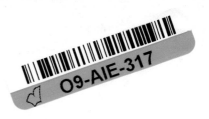

Managing Your Gestational Diabetes:

A Guide for You and Your Baby's Good Health

by Lois Jovanovic-Peterson, M.D.

With Morton B. Stone

JOHN WILEY & SONS, INC.

New York • Chichester • Weinheim • Brisbane • Singapore • Toronto

The information contained in this book is not intended to serve as a replacement for professional medical advice. Any use of the information in this book is at the reader's discretion. The author and the publisher specifically disclaim any and all liability arising directly or indirectly from the use or application of any information contained in this book. A health care professional should be consulted regarding your specific situation.

ISBN 0-471-34684-5

Printed in the United States of America

10   9   8   7   6

Table of Contents

Preface

The information in this book has a number of sources. Some of the information is based on my own experiences as a person who has diabetes and on my experiences during two pregnancies.

Other information stems from my 15 years of experience providing medical care to more than 500 pregnant women with diabetes. More than half of these women were diagnosed as having gestational diabetes.

Finally, a significant portion of the information in this book is derived from the findings of health care professionals throughout the world who have developed the tools and techniques of modern diabetes management.

A big thank you to my loving husband, Dr. Charles M. Peterson for supporting me through "our" diabetes and to Kevin, Larisa, and Boyce, who love me anyway.

Lois Jovanovic-Peterson, M.D.

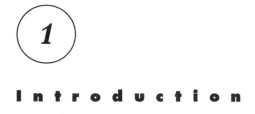

Introduction

If your physician has just told you that you have gestational diabetes or are at high risk for developing gestational diabetes, you're probably feeling frightened and upset. Maybe you've never heard of this disorder. And chances are you don't have any symptoms.

Gestation is another word for pregnancy, and gestational diabetes means the mother's body is not properly handling the glucose (sugar) from the food she eats. But why and how did this happen? What happens now? What are the risks for the baby?

No doubt you have many questions. That's good! It means you're beginning to cope with the problem. You want to be in control.

This book is designed to answer your questions about gestational diabetes. It provides information on what you need to do during your pregnancy and after, as well as some tips on how to ensure your good health in the years ahead.

If you still have questions after reading this book, be sure to ask your doctor, nurse, dietitian, diabetes educator, or counselor. They can—and should—answer all your questions about diabetes and its management. And the answers should be in words you can understand. If you don't clearly understand, please be sure to speak up and ask for clarification.

Once you've accepted the fact you have or are at risk for gestational diabetes, you may be ready to learn more about diabetes, in general, and gestational diabetes, in particular. The more you know, the better able you'll be to manage the remaining months of your pregnancy. With the help of your health care team, you'll be able to take the steps needed to control your gestational diabetes, reduce your own health risks—and, most important, protect your baby. To do this, you will have to make some lifestyle changes immediately and continue these through the remaining months of your pregnancy—and beyond.

- You will have to follow a special meal plan.

- You will have to monitor blood glucose.

- You may be required to inject a hormone called insulin every day.

- You may need to follow a regular exercise program.

Each of these activities will require some energy, time, and money. But the costs, time, and energy you spend now will ensure a healthy baby and a trouble-free delivery.

Although the information in this book is targeted toward you, it will be extremely beneficial to share this book with your husband or partner. He needs to know what you need to do, when you need to do it, and why it is so important to control gestational diabetes. Once he understands these things, he will be better able to support and help you during the next few months.

Finally, you may want to share the information in this book with other family members or close friends who are interested in your welfare. Friends and relatives are important members of your support team. And they, too, can benefit from the lifestyle changes discussed here—even if they don't have diabetes.

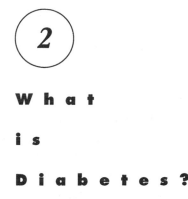

2

What

is

Diabetes?

Unlike other types of diabetes—which last a lifetime—gestational diabetes almost always goes away when you give birth.

Let's take a look at what diabetes is, what causes it, and how it is treated.

The complete scientific name for diabetes is *diabetes mellitus*. That's the umbrella for a group of diseases that have something in common—the inability of the body to properly use the glucose (sugar) provided by food. The three most common types of diabetes are type I, or insulin-dependent diabetes, type II, or noninsulin-dependent diabetes mellitus, and gestational diabetes.

Gestational Diabetes

Nobody knows the exact number, but most experts say between 3 and 12 percent of pregnant women develop gestational diabetes. That could be as many as half a million woman, which makes gestational diabetes the most frequently occurring metabolic disorder in pregnancy. In more than 85 percent of cases, the diabetes can be controlled by diet and exercise.

Gestational diabetes usually shows up in the last half of the pregnancy—from the 24th week onward. The condition develops at
this time because that is when the mother's body must greatly
increase the amount of nourishment provided to the growing
baby. At the same time, the levels of placental hormones peak,
and these hormones appear to weaken the effects of insulin in the
mother's body.

Early in pregnancy, while your baby is very small, extra nourishment isn't needed. But as your baby grows, the need for nourishment increases.

As you know, glucose provides the basic nourishment for your
body. The same holds true for your baby. Although you can eat
extra food to obtain additional nourishment, your baby is depen-
dent on you to break the food down into glucose. Glucose then
passes from your blood through the umbilical cord and placenta
to the fast-growing baby.

To meet your baby's needs for nourishment, your body must
produce an ever increasing supply of insulin. This is the hormone
that enables glucose to move from the bloodstream into the cells.
If you don't produce enough insulin, or if the insulin you produce doesn't work properly, your blood glucose will rise. High
blood glucose levels are harmful for the growing fetus. During
pregnancy, particularly in the second half, your insulin needs are
two to three times higher than when you were not pregnant.

Scientists do not yet know what causes gestational diabetes, but
in some women pregnancy seems to cause changes that interfere

• • • • • • • • • • • • • • • • •

with the way insulin works. Your body may not be able to produce sufficient amounts of insulin to handle the extra demand required during the second half of your pregnancy.

Or your body, particularly your placenta, may be producing hormones that interfere with the insulin you do produce. Your body reacts to this situation by producing more and more insulin and by releasing more and more glucose (which is stored in the liver). The end result is that glucose piles up in the bloodstream because it can't be used up by your body.

Excess glucose eventually is processed by your kidneys and spilled into your urine. But for the most part, the excess glucose stays in your bloodstream. Large amounts of glucose in your bloodstream over years may damage blood vessels and nerves and interfere with the normal functions of many of your body's vital organs.

Most physicians routinely test for gestational diabetes between the 24th and 28th weeks of pregnancy with a sugar drink. If this test shows that glucose levels are above normal, your doctor then does another test to determine just how your body handles even more sugar or carbohydrates (the major source of glucose). The doctor can then confirm whether or not you have a carbohydrate (sugar, glucose) intolerance—or what we call gestational diabetes.

Who's At Risk?

Because the exact causes of gestational diabetes aren't known, it's hard to know who is at greatest risk for this form of diabetes. However, medical textbooks point to some factors that occur more often than others in women with this disorder.

These factors include:

—a family history of diabetes

—a previous stillbirth

—a previous birth in which the baby weighed more than 9 pounds

—obesity, usually meaning more than 20 percent over ideal weight

—high blood pressure (hypertension)

—a history of skin, genital, or urinary tract infections

—a twin or triplet pregnancy

—age over 25

That last one seems as though it includes almost everyone and thus probably brings a huge number of women into the risk category. And that's exactly why routine screening is so important.

Is any one factor more important than than the others? No one knows for sure. Your doctor might say weight is the single most important factor, but even that is disputed. Whatever the cause, it's important to bear in mind that you didn't do anything to bring this on. Gestational diabetes affects women who are in great physical shape just as it hits those of us who weigh more than we should.

Routine Screening and Diagnostic Tests

Gestational diabetes can be difficult to recognize because there are usually no easily recognized symptoms. Fatigue, the need to urinate more often, and thirst are common in most pregnancies, so while these are classic symptoms of diabetes, pregnant women tend to see them as normal. The American Diabetes Association now recommends that all women who are pregnant be routinely screened for gestational diabetes.

In the past, a urine sugar test was used to screen for gestational diabetes. Now, however, more sophisticated tests are available. The first step is a screening blood glucose test, which you probably have already had. You drink a glass of very sweet liquid, then wait one hour, then have your blood tested. If the blood contains a high level of glucose, you need to have another test a few days later. If the blood glucose is normal or low at this first test, however, you can be pretty well assured you don't have gestational diabetes at this point.

The second test is called a glucose tolerance test. It's a longer version of the first. Before the test, you will be asked to eat a lot of carbohydrates—breads, cereals, rice, pasta, potatoes, etc.—which will help your body deal with what health professionals call a "glucose challenge." Your doctor or someone on your health care team should provide you with detailed instructions. You will then be told not to eat or drink anything but water after dinner on the night before the test.

Testing is usually done first thing in the morning. A sample of your blood is drawn as a "fasting sample," meaning you haven't had any food for fourteen or so hours. Then you will drink another glucose drink, this one bigger than the one you had at the first test. Your blood will then be tested each hour for the next three hours.

If the tests show abnormally high amounts of glucose for at least two of the total four readings, you have gestational diabetes. It is possible to have a high reading at the screening test and then have normal results with the glucose tolerance test. In fact, some studies show that 2 in 10 women will have positive screening tests, but only 1 in 4 of those with positive tests will actually have gestational diabetes.

If you are at a higher than normal risk for developing gestational diabetes, you may have to have a glucose tolerance test earlier than the 24th week. This is usually the case for women who have had gestational diabetes with a previous pregnancy.

When gestational diabetes is diagnosed later in your pregnancy, it is still important to do everything you can to safeguard your baby and your own health. Also, the risk for gestational diabetes increases as a woman gets older. Even though you didn't have it in an early pregnancy, you could get it with later ones.

What Are the Risks for the Baby?

With careful management, gestational diabetes seldom causes permanent effects for the baby. The catch is the careful management. You need to do exactly as your doctor, dietitian, or other health professionals advise.

Even though most babies are fine after gestational diabetes, there is a higher-than-normal risk for some complications. While we don't want to frighten you, you probably would feel better knowing exactly what any potential risks might be. So we'll explain them. Please keep in mind that these complications tend to be problems for women with poorly controlled gestational diabetes.

Macrosomia—This term means "large body" and refers to a baby who is larger than normal for its developmental age. Mothers who have high blood glucose levels are more likely to have very large babies. Before birth, the baby gets its "food" from the mother's blood supply, by way of the placenta. If more nourishment is available than the baby needs to grow normally, the excess is stored as fat. So high levels of sugar in the mother's blood can turn into large amounts of fat on the baby.

Hypoglycemia (low blood glucose)—This occurs at the time of birth if the baby's pancreas is making extra insulin to handle the high sugar in the mother's blood. After delivery, when the baby isn't getting glucose from the mother anymore, the extra insulin causes the baby's own blood glucose levels to fall too low. Then the baby might need to be given a glucose drink or an intravenous infusion of glucose.

Jaundice—This is a yellowing of the skin caused by a waste product named bilirubin. Babies need a large supply of red blood cells as they are growing inside the mother's womb. At birth, however, the baby no longer needs this extra supply, and the baby's body (specifically the liver) breaks down and gets rid of the old red cells. These broken-down cells are called bilirubin.

If the baby's liver isn't mature enough, it can't break down the red cells properly, and the bilirubin is left in the baby's tissues. Bilirubin makes the skin look yellow.

Many babies are born with a small amount of bilirubin, but if the amounts are higher than normal, special treatment may be needed. Usually this means placing the baby under special lights that help break down and get rid of the bilirubin. Very high levels of bilirubin can be dangerous for the baby and may require an exchange transfusion.

Jaundice in the baby can be a problem with gestational diabetes if the baby grows too quickly and must be delivered early. The chances that the liver won't be able to handle the red cells are then increased.

Respiratory distress syndrome (RDS)—This is a condition where the baby's lungs aren't developed enough for the baby to breathe on its own. RDS is always a risk for babies born prematurely. These babies usually need to be cared for in an intensive care unit until the lungs mature.

Risks for the Mom

Premature labor and delivery—These are more common with gestational diabetes than for other pregnancies. You probably will be closely monitored to detect and stop early labor. Sometimes this can mean having to stop work and maybe even going on bedrest toward the end of pregnancy. Also, cesarean deliveries are more common for women with gestational diabetes, partly to avoid problems if the baby is large.

Toxemia—Women with gestational diabetes have an increased risk for toxemia and urinary tract infections. Toxemia (also called preeclampsia) is the name for pregnancy-induced high blood pressure. It is often accompanied by swelling, usually in the feet and lower legs. High blood pressure is dangerous for both you and your baby. Treatment varies from limiting activity to hospitalization. Be sure to follow your health care team's advice!

Urinary tract infections—These seem to be more common in women with gestational diabetes than in other pregnant women. A burning sensation on urination and the feeling that you need to urinate often—sometimes all the time—are important symptoms. Be sure you let your health care team know if you have these problems. Antibiotics usually work to stop the infection. Ask your doctor if there's anything you can do to prevent later infections.

Ketones—These are acids produced when the mother's body breaks down fat because there is no other source of energy available. During pregnancy, this often means you aren't eating enough for both you and your baby.

Ketones are monitored because they can move through the placenta and into your baby's blood. Large amounts may be harmful to your baby. To be safe, you may be told to check your urine for ketones every morning. Your doctor can show you how this simple test works. Be sure you understand how often to test and when to notify your doctor if ketones are high.

To avoid this problem, it's important that you not skip meals or cut back on the number of calories you're eating. Pregnancy should never be a time for weight-loss or dieting.

Diabetes itself—If you have gestational diabetes once, you're likely to have it again with additional pregnancies. In addition, you have a high risk (between 25 and 60 percent) of developing permanent diabetes later in life.

Many experts believe this tendency to develop diabetes is inherited and little can be done about it. But there are some things you can do to prevent this, including careful weight control, good exercise habits, and good nutrition. We'll tell you more about these throughout this book.

Remember that bringing a healthy baby into the world is just the beginning of a lifelong commitment to caring for that child. You must, therefore, take the best possible care of yourself to ensure a healthy childhood for your new baby.

What Do You Need to Do to Control Your Blood Glucose?

Bringing your blood glucose levels into the normal range and keeping them there throughout the remaining days of your pregnancy is going to require making some changes. The rewards are great, though, so try not to be discouraged.

Meals and exercise are an important part of your plan. You must also monitor your blood glucose, keep records of your results, and see your doctor more often.

You will certainly need to spend time learning about your diabetes control program. For example, you probably want to:

- **Learn all that you can about diabetes in general and gestational diabetes in particular.** Reading this book is a good step.

- **Learn how to manage your gestational diabetes.** You'll need training from your doctor's diabetes educator (or the educator your doctor recommends) on the whys, whats, and how-to's of diabetes management.

- **Learn how to purchase and prepare foods that are included in your diabetes meal plan** (and to avoid foods that may upset your blood glucose balance). Remember, your diabetes meal plan is basically a good, healthy eating plan—one that can easily be followed by other members of your family.

- **Learn how to administer insulin injections, if your doctor prescribes them.** You'll also learn when and where to inject insulin and how to adjust your insulin dose when your blood glucose levels are too high or too low.

- **Learn how to measure your blood glucose levels.** Easy-to-use blood glucose meters are available to help you do this. But you must learn how to properly use the blood glucose meter and obtain a blood sample from your fingertip.

- **Learn how and when to exercise in a way that is safe for you and that will help improve your glucose control.**

- **Learn how to recognize certain diabetes-related problems that may occur** (such as low blood glucose) and how to respond to these problems.

Once you've learned these things, you need to put them into practice immediately. But we hope the healthy lifestyle you'll be living now will become a permanent one.

More About Diabetes

Many people don't realize there are three kinds of diabetes— type I, type II, and gestational. You've already learned a good deal about the gestational form, so we'll just briefly review the other types for you.

Type I Diabetes

This is the diabetes that attracts the most attention—primarily because it usually develops in youngsters and because it is life-threatening if not treated properly and effectively.

People with type I diabetes have lost the ability to produce any insulin. They require insulin injections in order to live.

Scientists believe this type of diabetes may develop slowly and silently over a period of years. For one or more reasons, the person's body develops antibodies to the cells that normally produce insulin, and then these antibodies slowly destroy the insulin-producing cells. Usually there are no symptoms of diabetes during this slow development period. But sophisticated tests can detect this process. Scientists are testing techniques that may be able to stop or slow the progression of the destructive process.

For most people, however, type I diabetes shows up suddenly and dramatically with severe symptoms. This occurs when the destructive process reaches a point where the body no longer is producing enough insulin to handle the glucose from foods. At this time, the person must use injected insulin to replace the insulin formerly produced by the body.

There are no known risk factors (other than a slight pattern of genetic inheritance) for type I diabetes. The disease usually strikes children, but it also can develop later in life. Although many people with type I may be thin, others are overweight. There is no link between pregnancy, even pregnancy complicated by gestational diabetes, and the development of type I diabetes.

People who have type I diabetes must follow a strict schedule of eating (with a prescribed meal plan), exercising (on a regular schedule), and self-blood glucose monitoring. Monitoring is important because it provides information for modifying treatment so blood glucose levels can be maintained in a normal range.

People with type I diabetes must inject insulin every day. The schedule usually is designed to meet their lifestyle and their diabetes needs. Recent scientific findings confirm that multiple injections (3 or 4 a day) along with a strict control program can prevent, delay, and reduce severity of diabetes complications. In addition to the usual needle-and-syringe injection method, a needleless spray injector or an insulin pump can be used. The pump infuses insulin into the body at a preset rate throughout the day and night, much like a normal pancreas would.

At present, there is no cure for type I diabetes. Scientists throughout the world are studying ways to interrupt the process of insulin-cell destruction that marks the beginning of this type of diabetes. Also, work is being done on improving techniques to transplant insulin-producing cells or the pancreas, where insulin-producing cells are located.

Type II Diabetes

The most common type of diabetes is type II, noninsulin-dependent diabetes (also called NIDDM, or adult-onset diabetes). More than 85 percent of all people who have diabetes have this type—including women who have had gestational diabetes. Most of these people still produce insulin, but their bodies cannot properly use the insulin, or they can't produce enough to meet their body's glucose needs. When either of these things happen, unused glucose piles up in the bloodstream and causes all sorts of problems.

Type II diabetes usually develops in people who are over the age of 40, are overweight, or have blood relatives with diabetes. Women who have delivered very large babies and those who have had gestational diabetes also are at an increased risk for developing type II diabetes.

The treatment for type II diabetes starts with a diabetes meal plan and exercise program designed to bring blood glucose levels back into the normal range. If excess weight is a problem, then the program is designed to reduce weight and keep it at normal. Even a small weight loss (10 percent of the body weight) can bring blood glucose levels back to normal and reduce symptoms for some people.

If the diet and exercise program isn't effective, then the person with type II diabetes probably will be given an oral antidiabetes medicine. (These drugs are dangerous for an unborn baby and therefore *cannot* be used during pregnancy.) Even with medication, the person with type II diabetes needs to stay with a diabetes meal plan and a regular exercise program. Also, a regular schedule of self-blood glucose monitoring is needed to check on how well the program is working.

Over a period of time, the oral medication, diet, and exercise program may lose effectiveness. The next step is to introduce a schedule of insulin injections (alone or in combination with the oral agent).

The objective of any treatment plan for diabetes is to normalize blood glucose and thus prevent, delay, or lessen the severity of diabetes-related complications later on. With gestational diabetes, your blood sugars are high for just a few months. With the other types of diabetes, high blood sugars over a number of years may cause kidney disease, circulation problems, and even blindness. You are the only person who can prevent this.

Types of Diabetes

	Type I (insulin dependent)	Type II (noninsulin dependent)	Gestational
Onset	Usually in children or young adults.	Usually in obese adults over age 40.	Occurs in 3 to 12% of pregnant women.
Cause	Inherited and other factors lead to failure of pancreas' ability to produce insulin.	Inherited tendency plus obesity leads to resistance of body cells to action of insulin.	Unknown, but hormonal and other changes may lead to high blood glucose.
Symptoms	Extreme thirst and excessive appetite, tiredness, and urination. May progress to ketoacidosis.	May be no obvious symptoms, or just slight fatigue, frequent thirst, and frequent urination.	Usually none. Fatigue, thirst, and excessive urination may occur but can be easily overlooked.
Diagnosis	Blood glucose test.	Glucose tolerance test.	Blood glucose screen followed by glucose tolerance test.
Treatment	Meal planning, exercise, and insulin injections.	Meal planning, exercise, and usually diabetes pills or sometimes insulin injections.	Meal planning, exercise, and sometimes insulin injections.

What Are You Feeling?

Suddenly learning you have a risky pregnancy can trigger all sorts of feelings—anger, guilt, depression, denial, fear. These are common feelings; everyone has them now and then. With your gestational diabetes, however, you need to be aware that feelings can sometimes get in the way of taking care of yourself.

Pregnancy is difficult for many women. The added stress of gestational diabetes can be more than some women can handle. Thinking about your feelings may help you cope with problems and deal with them appropriately.

Emotions sometimes become unhealthy—that is, they get in the way of what you need to do. For example, if you deny your gestational diabetes for a while, you can set yourself and your baby up for future problems. Similarly, fear can cause so much stress that it triggers high blood pressure or anxiety attacks.

The factors that affect whether an emotion will interfere with your life are its intensity—how strong it is—and its duration— how long it lasts. For example, guilt may be a problem for you, but only for a short time, until your rational mind can talk your irrational self out of fixing blame. Depression can be a short-term feeling, or it can last weeks. You need to be aware of how strong your feelings are and whether or not you have them for an unusually long time.

Every woman reacts differently to a diagnosis of gestational diabetes, and health professionals expect that you may experience some difficult feelings. They are concerned about extremes, however, and need to learn from you when you feel overwhelmed or unable to cope with your health.

With all types of diabetes, we usually think of certain feelings as normal but potentially troublesome.

They are:

Anger—

"Why me?" "This just isn't fair!" You're likely to feel angry at times because of the added stress and strain diabetes adds to your pregnancy. And some of that anger is healthy. It can energize you to deal with the problem—but it can't make your diabetes go away. Anger becomes unhealthy when it is misdirected—when we take it out on ourselves by not doing what needs to be done or when we take it out on people around us who have nothing to do with its cause.

Guilt—

This is very common with gestational diabetes because we tend to feel responsible for whatever happens. Here again, some guilt is healthy and useful. It can help get us back on the right road, doing what we must do each and every day. Blaming yourself, though, or thinking of yourself as "bad" or a "failure" is destructive. Remember, nothing you did or did not do caused you to have gestational diabetes. The main point now is to take good care of yourself.

Depression and sadness—

Feeling alone and misunderstood tend to alienate us from the very people who can help us most. You have come to recognize that you must deal with your diabetes, but you are very sad about the situation. Recognizing and accepting these feelings helps you adjust to your new lifestyle. When you're sad, you sometimes can make the changes in your self-image that help you cope with new challenges. You often think about the changes you must make and how life will be different. With healthy sadness, you usually learn to accept your situation.

Depression becomes unhealthy when it lasts too long and drains us of energy, causes a loss of appetite, or leads to sleeping problems. Isolation can make you feel worse and can lead to feelings of helplessness and hopelessness. Don't let this happen. Enlist support from family, friends, co-workers, and your health care team. They want to be there for you.

Denial—

"But I don't feel any different. This can't be happening to me." We all want to avoid the unpleasant and scary thoughts that come with some problems. And this can be healthy—at first. It protects you from other confusing feelings that can overwhelm you. It gives you a little cushion of time to get used to the idea of making changes in your life.

Without denial we would probably live in constant fear. But we can't deny an illness, particularly gestational diabetes, for very long. Recognize that some denial is normal as you learn to understand the problem, but then move on to taking the best care you possibly can of your baby and yourself.

Fear—

We all carry some fear all the time. Gestational diabetes triggers lots of fears, especially for the health and well-being of your child. But fear, too, can be a positive emotion if it motivates you to do what your doctor recommends. Appropriate fear, which represents an appropriate respect for consequences, can encourage you to be especially careful. On the other hand, too much fear can immobilize you and nurture a sense of helplessness. If you have strong fears, talk about them, especially with your health care team. They usually can reassure you and offer options for dealing with the fear and overcoming it.

And finally acceptance—

The last stage in working through your feelings about gestational diabetes is acceptance. You can come to terms with what needs to be done—and do it. Each person is unique, and we can't say how long it will take to accept changes you need to make. With gestational diabetes, however, you need to strive toward acceptance very early on.

Acceptance can lead to some very positive changes in your life. You can feel proud that you are coping with a difficult situation. You can feel in control—in charge. And you can come to recognize that you're capable of handling gestational diabetes without undue stress.

It's difficult to struggle with troubling feelings alone. Support from others can be crucial. If you are having a hard time dealing with your feelings, you need to ask for support from family, friends, and your health care team. If you still are troubled, you might be wise to get help from a professional counselor, social worker, or psychologist. These people are specially trained in dealing with difficult feelings and helping you learn how to express them in a healthy way.

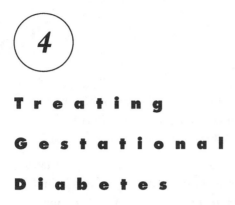

Treating Gestational Diabetes

The success of the treatment plan for controlling gestational diabetes hinges on your willingness to be an active participant in the program. You have total responsibility for eating the foods you and your baby need, for exercising on your prescribed schedule, for monitoring your blood glucose levels, and for taking your insulin injections (if prescribed) at the right time and in the right dose.

This is a big responsibility. But you have lots of people who can help you with the program. Unfortunately, they can't do it for you.

Your doctor can't give you your daily insulin shots. Your dietitian can't buy, prepare, and feed you foods on your meal plan. Your spouse can't exercise for you. And your friends can't do blood glucose measurements for you.

All of these people, however, can **help** you to do these things.

Blood Glucose Goals

For pregnant women who do not have gestational diabetes, blood glucose levels stay within a range of 60 to 120 milligrams per deciliter (mg/dl) (3.3 to 6.7 millimols per liter [mmol/L]).

They usually are 60 to 80 mg/dl (3.3 to 4.4 mmol/L) when measured after a period of fasting (such as first thing in the morning) and less than 120 mg/dl (6.7 mmol/L) after eating a meal.

For women with gestational diabetes, the goal is to keep fasting blood glucose levels at approximately 80 mg/dl (4.4 mmol/L) and at or under 120 mg/dl (6.7 mmol/L) after eating a meal.

Since you are reading this book, we hope you're ready to learn about what you need to do and how to do it.

The goal of any treatment plan for gestational diabetes is to keep your blood glucose levels within a normal range. If you do that, your risks for problems are significantly reduced.

When your blood glucose is above normal, there are a number of things you can do—some good, some not so good.

First, you can fast and thereby lower the quantity of glucose that enters your bloodstream. However, fasting will deprive your baby of the nutrients he or she needs for growth and development. Because of this, fasting is not recommended.

Second, you can reduce the amount of food you eat by cutting down on high-sugar, high-fat, and high-calorie snacks and meals and by eating smaller portions. This approach is okay if you also can maintain a properly balanced nutritional mix of carbohydrates, proteins, fats, vitamins, and minerals. If you reduce your food intake but maintain a nutritional balance, then your blood glucose levels should fall.

A diabetes meal plan developed by a dietitian is designed to do that for you. If you are overweight (in addition to the pounds you gained during the first half of your pregnancy), your diabetes meal plan also may be designed to prevent you from gaining additional, harmful pounds. You may even lose a little weight in the process. But it may be better for you to plan to drop your prepregnancy excess weight after you deliver your baby and then keep those pounds off in the future.

We'll provide more details about diabetes meal planning later in this book.

The next part of your treatment plan is *an exercise program* that will improve both your physical fitness and your blood glucose control. Exercise burns up calories (glucose) and thus directly reduces blood glucose levels. Exercise, combined with a reduced-calorie, balanced diet, can help you lose weight. Exercise also firms up and strengthens flabby muscles, and improves blood circulation. Exercise also can improve your emotional status. (Most people get a good feeling from regular exercise.)

There are some risks with exercise, so you need to listen to your body and exercise carefully and gently. Be especially careful in hot weather. And of course don't try any new, strenuous aerobic programs or fancy downhill skiing. A brisk walk after a meal might be perfect. But be sure to check with your doctor. Sometimes he or she will want you to use only your upper body when exercising toward the end of your pregnancy.

An essential part of your diabetes management program is a procedure called *self-blood glucose monitoring*. This procedure was not available to people with diabetes until a little more than a decade ago. The development of easy-to-use, relatively inexpensive, and accurate blood glucose meters allows people with diabetes to check their blood glucose levels at home, at work, or anywhere else and at any time they choose.

The process allows you to see precisely what your blood glucose levels are at the time of the measurement. And testing only takes a minute or so to do. The results of the glucose measurement provide you and members of your diabetes care team with valuable information that can be used to fine-tune your control program.

- You can use self-blood glucose monitoring to find out how your body reacts to certain foods—to see how a portion of a specific food increases your blood glucose.

- You can use self-blood glucose monitoring to see how exercise affects your blood glucose levels.

- You can see what a minor illness (such as a cold) or a stressful situation does to your blood glucose levels.

- You can see how an insulin injection (if this is prescribed) works to lower your blood glucose levels. You can see whether the "under the weather" feelings you have are caused by abnormal blood glucose levels or if they are caused by an upcoming storm or visit from the in-laws.

Your doctor will develop a schedule for you to follow for blood glucose monitoring. Your doctor or diabetes educator will also teach you how to use the blood glucose monitoring system you select. (There are many to choose from.)

Finally, you'll learn how to record results and other vital facts and how and when you should make adjustments in your diet, exercise, and medication if your blood glucose levels are not in the normal range.

More information on blood glucose monitoring and other types of tests will be provided as you continue through this book.

Insulin Injections

You may require insulin injections to keep your blood glucose levels in a normal range. Your doctor will determine this, based on the results of the initial diagnostic blood tests and the success or lack of success you have with managing your gestational diabetes with diet and exercise alone.

If you need insulin, you may only need one injection before breakfast each day or perhaps before bed. But, in some cases, three or four injections may be needed each day.

Multiple injections of insulin have a great advantage over a single injection because more frequent insulin injections more closely mimic the natural production and release of insulin. It's not the same as the natural, but it comes as close as it can without use of an insulin pump, which releases a set amount of insulin on a continuous basis.

If you need insulin, your blood glucose monitoring will be scheduled so you can see how the combination of food and insulin balances.

The insulin and the insulin delivery devices available to you far surpass those used even a few years ago. You may use "human" insulin that is manufactured but is exactly like the insulin the human body produces. Use of human insulin reduces the risks of allergic reactions and developing resistance, which were common when insulin was obtained from the pancreas glands of pigs and cows.

Modern needles and syringes are virtually painless to use and more convenient to handle and dispose of.

Your doctor or diabetes educator will teach you how and where to inject insulin and will set up a schedule that provides guidelines for when and how much insulin to inject.

More information about insulin is given in the chapters that follow.

Ongoing Care, Checkups, and Tests

You are now about to embark on a program that will carry you through the remaining months of your pregnancy. This will be a very important time for you and for your baby. Your health care professionals will be there at every step to support you, help you, and answer your questions.

One thing these health professionals cannot do is perform the tasks needed to keep your gestational diabetes in good control and to ensure both your own and your baby's health.

Your first step is to have a comprehensive diabetes plan designed for you. You'll need to rely on your doctor to handle the medical aspects of the plan. Your diabetes educator will teach you how to implement all aspects of the plan (such as how to monitor blood glucose, inject insulin, and handle emergencies). You need the expertise of your dietitian to design a meal plan for you and to help you modify this meal plan when needed. You need a member of the health care team to advise you about how and when to exercise safely.

Your next step is to stay in close touch with members of the team during the next few months. Visits to your doctor's office will be stepped up, first to as frequently as you need to learn the program, then to approximately every two weeks, and then to once a week.

Not only will your glucose levels be checked at these office visits, but also your doctor may do nonstress tests, contraction stress tests, or other tests to determine if the baby's growth and development are going according to plan. Each time you visit the doctor, you will be asked to bring along your diabetes record book, which should contain information about your food intake, blood glucose measurements, medication dosage, exercise, and other facts. If you have some unanswered questions, write these down before your visit and then get the answers from your doctor or another member of your health care team.

If you and your doctor have agreed to have elective delivery, meaning either a cesarean section or induced labor, other tests may need to be done, such as amniocentesis and ultrasound. (Don't worry. We'll tell you about these tests later).

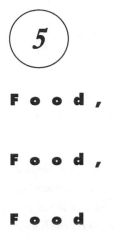

Food,

Food,

Food

Marilyn was thrilled to learn she, indeed, was pregnant. She and her husband went out to their favorite restaurant and celebrated by eating a seven course meal, complete with wine and a yummy dessert cake. The cake was so good, Marilyn even finished off her husband's portion.

Although this was a very special evening, it was quite similar to the fun-filled ones she enjoyed throughout much of her adult life (before and after marriage). She felt that life was to be enjoyed along with food, song, and friendships. She dedicated many hours to such enjoyments and still more hours trying to fight the extra pounds she carried on her body since high school.

Once she learned she was pregnant, she believed she no longer had to watch calories. She followed her mother's advice: She now had to eat for two, and the extra pounds would provide extra nutrition for the growing baby.

By the middle of her pregnancy, she had gained 40 pounds.

At that time, her doctor gave her a routine simple blood glucose test, followed by another, more complicated battery of tests. The tests showed Marilyn had gestational diabetes.

The doctor referred her to a dietitian on the staff of the local hospital. After talking with Marilyn about her eating habits and preferences, the dietitian developed a specially designed meal plan—one that would help Marilyn control her weight and help to keep her blood glucose levels within a normal range.

The dietitian advised Marilyn how to calculate food exchanges and how to count calories. She discussed various food choices and how to substitute good-tasting, healthy foods for high-fat and high-sugar ones. She pointed out how food preparation techniques are important and how controlling portion sizes is essential for anyone concerned about weight.

Marilyn also learned she needed to measure her blood glucose levels one hour after each meal—to see how foods affected her blood glucose levels and also to confirm that the prescribed meal plan was keeping her blood glucose under good control.

Although it was difficult, Marilyn followed the meal plan through the last half of her pregnancy. The hard work paid off when she delivered a healthy baby girl, who arrived right on time and at the perfect weight.

You Are What You Eat

That saying is particularly appropriate for you now. You're eating for two and will do so for the remaining weeks of your pregnancy.

What you eat and when you eat will have a tremendous effect on you and your unborn child.

Consider this: **Food is the most important part of your effort to control gestational diabetes and ensure that you remain healthy and deliver a normal baby**. All other parts of your program hinge on your ability to choose the right kinds of food, eat the right amounts of food, and eat on a specific schedule.

Without the right kind of meal plan, your exercise program, your blood glucose monitoring, and even your insulin injection plan won't do anything to keep your blood glucose levels in the normal range. As a matter of fact, if you don't eat food at the right time and in the right amount, a session of exercise or an injection of insulin can send your blood glucose down to dangerous levels. This is called hypoglycemia, which is one of the short-term complications of all forms of diabetes.

Don't be misled by television commercials that promise a healthy diet in a can. That's not possible for you. Your diet must be designed for you, and you alone. Your body is different from other people's—even other people with diabetes. Your lifestyle, too, is different. This means your diabetes meal plan must be tailored to your body, your lifestyle, your diabetes, and your pregnancy.

Fortunately, your health care team, particularly the dietitian who has experience in developing diabetes meal plans, can help you develop an individualized gestational diabetes meal plan. You'll need to set aside some time to discuss the elements of the plan with the dietitian, who will want to know your food preferences and eating habits.

With this information, the dietitian can develop a meal plan that meets the recommendations of the American Diabetes Association, but is slightly modified to accommodate the special requirements of gestational diabetes. Your basic meal plan will include three meals and three snacks each day, with specific calorie quotas for each of these eating times.

To maintain your blood glucose within the normal range, your meal plan should provide the following:

• Breakfast: 10 to 15 percent of total daily calories

• Mid-morning snack: 5 to 10 percent of total daily calories

• Lunch: 30 percent of total daily calories

• Mid-afternoon snack: 5 to 10 percent of total daily calories

• Dinner: 30 percent of total daily calories

• Evening snack: 5 to 10 percent of total daily calories

In addition to calories, your personal meal plan will provide the carbohydrate, protein, fat, vitamins, and minerals you need each day.

The gestational diabetes meal plan usually includes 40 percent or less of calories from carbohydrates (preferably complex carbohydrates such as whole-wheat breads and cereals), 20 to 25 percent of calories from protein (preferably low-fat, lean meats, poultry, fish and beans or legumes); and 30 to 40 percent of calories from fats (preferably monounsaturated and polyunsaturated).

A sample menu for a gestational diabetes meal plan follows. This is just a guide. Your doctor and dietitian will put together a plan that is correct for you. Be sure to ask questions if you don't understand the meal plan or if you have concerns about how the plan fits your lifestyle.

Sample 1,800-calories menu
(40% of total calories are from carbohydrate)

Meal	Carbohydrate (grams)	Calories	Percent of calories from carbohydrate
Breakfast			
1 egg	0	100	
1 slice whole-wheat toast	15	80	
1 cup caffeine-free			
tea or coffee	0	0	
Total		**180**	**10%**
Mid-morning Snack			
1 medium apple	15	60	
1 ounce cheese	0	100	
Total		**160**	**10%**
Lunch			
2 slices whole-wheat bread	30	160	
2 ounces water-packed tuna	0	110	
Tossed green salad	10	50	
2 teaspoons mayonnaise	0	90	
Total		**410**	**20%**
Mid-afternoon Snack			
1 slice whole-wheat bread	15	80	
1 tablespoon sugar-free			
peanut butter	0	100	
1 glass caffeine-free iced tea	0	0	
Total		**180**	**10%**

Meal	Carbohydrate (grams)	Calories	Percent of calories from carbohydrate
Dinner			
4 ounces lean meat, fish, or poultry	0	220	
1 small baked potato	15	80	
1/2 cup steamed broccoli	0	0	
1/2 cup carrots	10	50	
1 piece fruit	15	60	
8 ounces skim milk	12	100	
1 whole-wheat roll	15	80	
3 teaspoons margarine	0	135	
Total		**725**	**40%**
Evening Snack			
8 ounces skim milk	12	90	
1 graham cracker	15	80	
Total		**170**	**10%**
Grand Total	**179**	**1825**	**100%**

In addition, your food selection should include lots of fiber-rich foods, such as vegetables, whole-grain breads, fruits (except at breakfast), and beans or legumes. Increased intake of fiber will help you maintain bowel regularity and may also help control your blood glucose levels.

This special meal plan most probably will require you to change your eating habits. First of all, you will need to eat a very small breakfast—one that does NOT include a glass of fruit juice or a portion of fresh fruit. You'll also need to severely limit your intake of breakfast breads and other high-carbohydrate foods. *This is the most important change you will have to make in your eating habits. Your body, particularly now when you have gestational diabetes, just cannot handle large amounts of carbohydrates in the morning without piling these carbohydrates up in your bloodstream as excess amounts of glucose.*

Next, your meal plan will include between-meal snacks. If you build your snack around a protein food, you will be able to avoid the extreme hunger that leads to overeating at the next meal. You'll also find that a plan that features smaller main meals and multiple snacks will help you digest foods better and easier and help you avoid uncomfortable heartburn.

The dietitian who designs your meal plan will teach you how to use the exchange system developed jointly by the American Diabetes Association and the American Dietetic Association for people who have diabetes.

Briefly, the exchange system is based on the amount of carbohydrate, protein, fat, and calories in each food. Similar foods are grouped together and can be "exchanged" with each other without changing the composition of the meal.

For example, if your meal plan calls for 2 bread or starch exchanges, you might choose 1 slice of toast and 1/2 cup of cereal. Or you could choose 1 cup of cereal and no toast or 2 English muffin halves and no cereal. You will be able to use the exchange system to determine what foods to include in each meal or snack and how to substitute one food for another one.

The dietitian also will recommend that you keep a daily record of the amount and type of foods you eat and the times you eat.

The information in the sample record book on page 111 will help you learn how to balance your food intake against the blood glucose readings you obtain from monitoring. The record book also should be used to record exercise sessions, blood glucose readings, and medication dosage and timing.

As part of your meal plan education, you'll learn how to estimate portion size and to determine calorie and nutrient content of the foods you eat. If you were overweight before you became pregnant, you probably have gained even more pounds during the past few months. Those extra pounds might have contributed to the development of gestational diabetes, and they may be making your task of normalizing your blood glucose much more difficult.

Should you restrict calorie intake to control your weight, or even lose excess pounds? Will restricting the amount of calories you eat harm or help your baby?

These are excellent questions. And the answers should ease your concerns.

Scientific studies have shown that a moderate restriction of calories in obese women with gestational diabetes does help prevent fetal macrosomia (excess birth weight). When you restrict your calorie intake, you may normalize the birth weight of your baby and you may also reduce your insulin needs. Calorie restriction at this stage in your pregnancy also will reduce the chances that you will be obese after delivery—and this will reduce your risks for developing diabetes in the future.

A word of caution: Don't go on a calorie-restricted diet (or a commercial quick weight-loss program) without the approval of your doctor. If you cut calories too much, you will be depriving your baby of the nutrients he or she needs for normal growth and development.

Your calorie-reduction program may not be totally designed to help you lose weight. You may have to wait until after you give birth to make this lifestyle change. But the program will help you to limit the amount of weight you gain during the last three months. Your doctor and dietitian will determine just how much weight you should gain during this period.

Keeping and Using Records

Record keeping provides valuable information that allows you and your health care team to fine-tune your diabetes management program. You can use a preprinted diabetes record book that has been modified by your dietitian to suit your pregnancy management plan. These books are available from a number of manufacturers and sold either through the mail or from your local diabetes association or diabetes center. We have included some sample pages at the back of this book. You can copy them if you like. Or you can put together your own diary—just as long as it includes spaces for you to record:

- Food intake at meals and snacks (amount and time)

- Blood glucose monitoring results (including time)

- Exercise sessions (type and length of time)

- Medication, if prescribed (time of insulin injection, dosage, and type of insulin)

- Plus any events in your life that day that may have interfered with your keeping to your diabetes management plan.

Your record book will help you and your health care team know whether or not your meal plan is working. The information on what you have eaten and when can be matched against the blood glucose readings you got after you finished eating. If your blood glucose level one hour after eating is less than 120 mg/dl (6.7 mmol/L), you know your meal plan is working. If the level is higher than 120 mg/dl (6.7 mmol/L), adjustments need to be made in the meal plan, your exercise program, or your medication dose and schedule.

Your records will also tell you if your body responds in a special way to certain foods. Sensitivity to some foods may send your blood glucose levels soaring out of the normal range.

Your record book can also help you keep track of the weight you are gaining on the prescribed meal plan. If the weight gain is not within preset goals, then adjustments need to be made.

Best of all, your record book will be your best teacher about how to make decisions on what and how much to eat. This decision-making ability gives you the power to control your life and your pregnancy.

Daily Food Quotas

Not only do you need to follow the basic dos and don'ts about when you should eat certain foods, but also you need to keep in mind that your body requires a balanced intake of fruits, vegetables, breads, starches, meat, fat, and calcium-rich dairy products. Here is a chart that can serve as a guideline to help you meet your daily nutritional needs.

Daily Nutritional Needs

	Servings each day*	Amount per serving	Suggestions
Milk	4 or more*	-8-ounce glass of skim or low-fat milk -1 cup of plain yogurt -1 ounce of low-fat cheese -1/4 cup skim-milk cottage cheese	If you don't like milk (or can't tolerate it) switch to low-fat cheeses or yogurt. Milk and milk products supply calcium, phosphorus, protein, and vitamins.
Vegetables	2 or more	-1/2 cup cooked -1 cup raw	Eat at least one serving of dark green or yellow vegetables (broccoli, spinach, greens, carrots, or winter squash). Vegetables supply both vitamins and minerals.

	Servings each day*	Amount per serving	Suggestions
Fruits	3 or more	–1/2 grapefruit –1 medium whole apple, lemon, lime, or tomato.	Choose one serving of citrus or other fruit high in vitamin C.
Breads & Cereals	4 or more	–1 slice bread –3 cups popcorn –1/2 cup cooked cereal, pasta, rice, or potatoes –3/4 cup packaged cereal	Select complex carbohydrate sources that contain whole grains and supply lots of fiber along with minerals, vitamins, and carbohydrates.
Meat	6 ounces	–1 ounce cooked meat, poultry, or fish –1 cup cooked beans, –1/2 cup cooked lentils –1 egg	Pregnancy demands extra ingestion of protein (about 30 grams a day). The 6 ounces of protein can be made up of 2 ounces of meat plus 6 cups of milk (4 from the milk group plus 2 extra cups).
Fat	3 or less	–1 teaspoon of margarine, oil, or mayonnaise	Select monounsaturated (olive oil) or polyunsaturated (corn oil) rather than saturated (hydrogenated shortening).

*The information in this chart should serve only as a guideline. Your individualized meal plan will provide you with specifics.

General Nutrition Tips

- Follow a regular eating schedule, trying to eat at the same time every day and keeping meals the same size. This is especially important if you need to inject insulin.

- Try to put your sweet tooth on vacation during your pregnancy. Avoid foods that contain simple sugars (such as table sugar). Also, avoid using excessive amounts of artificial sweeteners.

- Eat sufficient amounts of foods to provide a well-balanced intake of nutrients and enough calories to either maintain your present weight or to provide for an appropriate weight gain needed to handle your pregnancy needs.

- Be careful about the kinds of foods you eat. Whenever possible, eat foods that contain lots of fiber (such as vegetables, whole-grain breads and cereals, and fresh fruits, except at breakfast). Be sure to drink lots of water when you increase your fiber intake.

- Watch out for fat, particularly saturated fat found in meat and dairy products. Select low-fat dairy products, lean cuts of meat, fish and poultry, and use low-fat methods of cooking (such as broiling, baking, steaming, and roasting).

- Take advantage of the free foods available to you to satisfy your appetite and not upset your meal plan (sugar-free beverages, decaffeinated tea or coffee, unsweetened gelatin). Your dietitian will explain which foods can be considered "free."

- Avoid alcohol.

- Avoid or reduce your intake of caffeine-rich foods, such as coffee, tea, and chocolate.

- Restrict salt intake if your doctor advises.

- Avoid spicy and greasy foods. Don't lay down right after you eat a meal. Eat slowly and be sure to chew your food well.

- Drink plenty of liquids (at least 8 glasses each day); drink some of these between meals, rather than with them.

- Get plenty of exercise. Your doctor will tell you the kind and amount best for you. Exercise will help you to look and feel better, to burn off calories, and to control your blood glucose levels.

Meal Plan Guidelines

- Avoid eating cookies, cakes, pies, regular soft drinks, chocolate, table sugar, fruit juices and drinks, and regular jams and jellies.

- Avoid eating "fast foods" and packaged, convenience foods such as instant noodles, canned soups, instant potatoes, frozen meals, and packaged stuffings and "helpers."

- Learn to read labels and then avoid (or substitute for) foods that are high in fat, salt, or sugar (by any name). Other commonly known sugars are corn syrup, honey, and molasses. Different sugars have names that end in "ose," such as fructose and galactose. Sugar alcohols have names that end in "ol," such as sorbitol and mannitol.

- Eat every three hours or so. Include a good source of protein in every meal or snack (try low-fat meat, chicken, turkey, fish, cheese; or nuts, peanut butter, or skim-milk cottage cheese).

- Eat a very small breakfast that contains a good protein source. Avoid fruits and fruit juices. Limit your starch/bread choice to one exchange at breakfast.

- Choose foods that are high in fiber, such as whole-grain breads and cereals, fruits (except at breakfast), beans, legumes, and vegetables.

- Try to lower your total intake of fat, with particular attention to saturated fat. Avoid deli or processed meats (hot dogs, salami, etc.). Choose low-fat cuts of beef and veal. Select fish and poultry often, particularly the white meat of chicken and turkey.

- Trim visible fat from meat and fish before cooking. Remove skin from poultry before eating. Skim fat off of stews, soups, and casseroles.

- Select cooking methods that don't use fat (broil, bake, roast, or steam rather than fry or sauté). If you must sauté, use a nonstick pan and vegetable spray instead of oil.

- Choose vegetable oils (such as canola, corn, or olive) rather than hydrogenated shortenings and butter.

- Use skim or low-fat milk and dairy products.

- Avoid adding fat to your diet in the form of butter, sour cream, cream cheese, and regular mayonnaise, or salad dressings. Plain nonfat yogurt makes a good substitute, especially for dips and salad dressing.

- Eat any quantity of the following free foods at any time you desire: cabbage, cucumbers, green onions, mushrooms, zucchini, spinach, celery, green beans, radishes, and lettuce. All of these can be eaten raw or combined in a salad or soup.

6

Exercise

Carol was first diagnosed as having gestational diabetes by her obstetrician and was referred to our diabetes center for specialized care. She had lots of questions and expressed fear for her own health as well as the health of her baby. She told us that she was interested in learning as much as she could about both diet and exercise. After an initial session to answer some of her many questions, she decided to enroll in the diet and exercise program offered by our diabetes center.

Carol's first exercise session ended after five minutes because she was too tired to continue. Even though her body let her down, her resolve was strong. She pledged she would come back for the next scheduled session.

She did—and she became so enthusiastic about exercise, she had to be told when each session was over. She continued to build up her strength and endurance until the program was concluded.

Not only did Carol get a new exercise wardrobe to work out in during her pregnancy, she also purchased a sleeker wardrobe so that she could continue her exercise "habit" after she gave birth—which she did on time and without complications—to a healthy baby girl.

Physical activity is an important part of your program to control your gestational diabetes. Exercise of the proper kind and proper amount can do a lot of good things for you.

In most women with gestational diabetes, an exercise program can help keep blood glucose levels under good control. Exercise not only burns off calories, but also it increases muscle tone, builds cardiovascular fitness, relieves tension and anxiety, and helps body cells become more sensitive to insulin, thereby overcoming insulin resistance.

Most women can do some form of exercise from the time they become pregnant until very nearly the time they feel their first labor pains. The fact that you have been diagnosed as having gestational diabetes does not mean you should stop exercising. It does, however, mean you need to select certain types of exercise and check with your diabetes care professional before starting any exercise program or if you experience any problems when you are exercising.

There are a few cautions that every pregnant woman should observe—and there are special recommendations for women who have gestational diabetes. Here are some general cautions:

- **Listen to your body**. If you feel fatigued when you exercise, stop what you are doing and rest your body. If you feel pain or discomfort, don't continue the activity. Check immediately with your diabetes care professional. If you have a minor illness (such as a cold), take a break from your exercise program. If you suffer a minor exercise-related injury, such as a strain or sprain, take a few days off and allow your body to heal itself. If your blood glucose measurements are out of the normal range—either too low, or too high—make sure you take steps to correct them (by either changing your insulin dosage or your food intake) **before** you start an exercise session.

- **Exercise in moderation.** Even if you were physically fit before you started your pregnancy, you need to cut down on the intensity of your exercises and even avoid certain activities that may put your body—and your baby—at risk. Your diabetes care professional probably will advise you to avoid physical activities that involve twists, turns, jumping, sudden starts and stops, and high-impact activities such as jogging. Wait until you deliver your healthy baby before you return to the racquetball, volleyball, and basketball courts. Be wise and cut out potentially dangerous activities such as water skiing and snow skiing.

- **Do not exercise without the approval of your doctor.** Take advantage of your doctor's expertise by checking with him or her about your exercise plans. You may be advised not to engage in a strenuous exercise program if you suffer from such health problems as anemia, heart disease, untreated thyroid disease, or high blood pressure (hypertension). Your doctor may prescribe a modified physical activity plan. You may also need a special exercise program if you are greatly overweight or underweight. Exercise may be severely restricted or even forbidden if you experience vaginal bleeding during your pregnancy or if you are at increased risk for premature labor.

If your doctor says you must restrict your physical activity to avoid premature labor or other complications, you may still be able to do upper-arm exercises—such as lifting two-pound weights while seated in a chair. You can do upper-arm exercises in the comfort of your home no matter what the weather is outside. You can do it while watching TV or even while meditating, to ease tension.

To get sufficient benefits, your upper-arm exercise sessions should run 15 to 30 minutes (you can split the total time into two sessions if you prefer). Exercise on a daily basis. If you feel too fatigued or under the weather, that day you can skip a session. But don't take a long vacation from exercise. You may find it difficult to get back into the exercise routine if you skip more than a day or two.

If you are injecting insulin to control your blood glucose, you need to be particularly alert to changes in your blood glucose levels. Both insulin and exercise will lower blood glucose levels. To avoid a low blood glucose attack, be sure to measure your blood glucose before and after exercise. If the level is below normal before you start exercise, eat a snack to bring your glucose levels up.

If this low level of blood glucose becomes the "norm," report your measurements to your doctor. This pattern may mean that your insulin dosage needs adjustment. It may also mean your hard work at exercising may be paying off by lowering your blood glucose levels.

A below-normal blood glucose measurement after exercise may mean one of two things: Either the exercise you did was too strenuous, or the insulin/meal combination before exercise was not adequate to "cover" the exercise session. Ask your diabetes care professional to advise you on adjustments if this happens to you.

Another form of exercise that may be okay for you is walking. A brisk walk for 20 to 30 minutes after you have eaten may be good for your digestion and for controlling your blood glucose levels.

One of the best times to include walking in your schedule is right after breakfast, when your blood glucose levels may be at their highest point of the day. As your pregnancy progresses, you may find it is more difficult to do extensive walking. That's when weight lifting while sitting in a chair becomes much more attractive—and practical.

Swimming can also be an excellent exercise choice. Many pregnant women find that water exercise eases stress on the joints, feet, and legs.

If this is not your first pregnancy and you have youngsters at home, you may be reaching your exercise quota just by providing routine care for them. But, even if you have lots of household chores, you need to set some time aside for your special exercise program.

In the days or weeks immediately before you give birth, your diabetes care professional may recommend that you ease off on your exercise program. Consider this only as a brief and temporary vacation from exercise.

After the Baby is Born

About four to six weeks after your baby is born, you need to get back into a regular exercise program. (Note: If you have a cesarean delivery, you may have to wait a bit longer before resuming your exercise program.)

There are many reasons for making exercise a part of your post-delivery life:

- Your need for physical fitness increases after the baby is born. The physical and emotional demands of caring for a newborn, as well as the rest of your family, will be significant. Physical activity will help you regain your prepregnancy shape. Exercise will tone up your muscles, help flatten your tummy, and increase your flexibility and endurance—which you'll need to keep up with the new addition to your family.

- The longer you wait after delivery to start an exercise program, the harder it will be to get back in shape.

- Exercise will help you to lose excess pounds that you put on during pregnancy. Exercise burns calories, and works best when combined with a calorie-restricted diet. If you were overweight to begin with or if you gained too many pounds during pregnancy, then an exercise/diet plan may be your best choice.

- Exercise helps control blood glucose levels. Your gestational diabetes may have gone away the minute you started labor, but your risks for developing type II diabetes in the future are increased. If you weigh more than is desirable after your pregnancy, you have about a 60 percent chance of developing type II diabetes. If you get your weight down and keep it down, the risk drops to 25 percent. By controlling blood glucose levels after pregnancy (and by losing excess pounds) you will reduce the chances that you will develop this type of diabetes in years to come.

Insulin

Martha has a strong family history of type II, noninsulin-dependent diabetes. Her mother, grandmother, and two aunts have it. Martha weighed more than 10 pounds at birth. Her mother developed gestational diabetes during the third trimester of pregnancy and later developed type II diabetes.

Martha's first two pregnancies were normal. In the middle of her third pregnancy, however, the routine screening test showed high glucose values. The oral glucose-tolerance test confirmed a diagnosis of gestational diabetes.

At first, Martha was advised to try to manage the gestational diabetes through a program of diet, exercise, and blood glucose monitoring. She adhered to the recommended program quite strictly. But, no matter how closely she kept to the program, her blood glucose levels remained above the normal range. It was obvious that the program was not working effectively, despite Martha's efforts.

Martha kept in close contact with her health care team, and after a very short time it was decided that Martha needed to add insulin injections to her diabetes management program. Her doctor prescribed injections three times a day. Her health care team members instructed her on how to inject insulin properly, and she started the new program. She saw the results within a few days, when her blood glucose levels returned to the normal range, and stayed there. The remaining eight weeks of her pregnancy were without problems and she delivered a healthy boy who was perfect in every way.

If your doctor has told you that you need insulin injections to control your gestational diabetes, you probably are experiencing a number of rather strong reactions.

- *You may be upset* because you have to inject yourself with a hypodermic needle and syringe and are afraid of not doing this right—or doing it at all.

- *You may be confused* because you have read that insulin injections are needed by people with severe, life-long diabetes, and your doctor has told you that your diabetes will probably go away when you give birth.

- *You may even be angry* because this terrible thing has happened to you and has further complicated your already complicated pregnancy.

These are legitimate feelings and concerns. But, with the help of your family, friends, and members of your health care team, you will in time be able to deal with them and even overcome most of these negative responses.

Here's something positive to consider: The insulin injections your doctor has prescribed will help you—and your baby—to stay healthy. Not long ago, the diagnosis of gestational diabetes carried with it a major concern for the health of the mother and a significantly increased risk for birth defects in the child. Insulin therapy, along with diet, exercise, and monitoring, changed the odds in favor of the mother and child.

Why Insulin Injections?

Although some women with gestational diabetes are able to effectively control their blood glucose levels by following a meal plan, exercise program, and monitoring schedule alone, other women just can't do this. For one or more reasons, these women require insulin injections to maintain good glucose control.

If diet, exercise, and monitoring do not maintain finger-stick blood glucose levels **consistently** below 90 mg/dl (5 mmol/L) fasting or 120 mg/dl (6.7 mmol/L) one hour after eating, then insulin injections are needed. (Note: If your doctor measures your blood glucose by drawing blood from your vein and sending it to a laboratory, these laboratory determinations are 105 [5.8 mmol/L] fasting and 140 [7.8 mmol/L] one hour after meals.)

A single reading that is too high or two low may be a chance occurrence. But two or more "abnormal" blood glucose readings within a week or so means something needs fixing. And that fixing, in most cases, is to start a program of insulin injections. If your doctor has said you need insulin injections, you will get training and support from a health care professional on your doctor's staff or at a local diabetes center. You will learn when to take insulin injections, how to inject insulin, when the insulin takes peak effect, and how long its effects last. You will learn to recognize the symptoms of low blood sugar, as well as how to prevent it and how to treat it if it occurs. You will also learn how and when to make adjustments in either your dosage of insulin, the amount or type of food you eat, or your exercise routine based on blood glucose measurements.

In most cases, instructions for managing your diabetes will take place at your doctor's office or at the outpatient clinic of a local diabetes center or hospital. If these services are not available to outpatients, you may need to be hospitalized for this process. Although diabetes care professionals may have different philosophies about there are some general guidelines.

Most women with gestational diabetes find that only their fasting blood glucose measurements are above normal. These women can usually keep their after-meal blood glucose levels normal with diet alone. When the diet approach doesn't work, however, then insulin injections are needed.

The first step is to have the woman inject a dose of insulin in the evening, just before bedtime. This usually is an intermediate-acting (8-hour) insulin called NPH. The starting dosage generally is 0.1 to 0.15 units for each kilogram of body weight. That means that if you are obese, a higher starting dosage of insulin is necessary. The dosage of insulin can then be increased gradually until the fasting blood glucose measurement drops below 90 mg/dl (5.0 mmol/L).

If after-meal blood glucose readings are above normal, too, then a more comprehensive insulin injection-program is needed. This requires injecting insulin three or, in some cases, four times a day. In addition to the intermediate-acting NPH insulin, a short-acting (Regular) insulin is added to the program. A typical three-injection program consists of an injection of NPH plus Regular before breakfast (2/3 of the total daily dose), an injection of Regular before dinner (1/6 of the total daily dose) and an injection of NPH at bedtime (1/6 of the total daily dose).

. . . .

Most doctors recommend that "human" insulin be used, rather than pork or beef insulin. The human insulin, which is manufactured but is virtually identical to that produced by the normal pancreas, is better tolerated and less likely to cause resistance or allergic reactions.

Your insulin dosage often will need to be increased as your pregnancy advances. This is because your body's resistance to the action of insulin also increases. You can keep track of these changes by regularly testing your glucose. When you see a pattern of high blood glucose readings, you will need to contact your health care professional about adjusting your dosage.

To keep your blood glucose control finely tuned, you'll have to take major responsibilities yourself. You will have to measure your blood glucose levels frequently and then make adjustments in your program (diet, exercise, and medication) when you see that your blood glucose is outside the normal range.

Call your health care professional if your blood glucose levels fall out of the normal range and you don't know what to do. Don't wait days or weeks to obtain face-to-face advice—your gestational diabetes won't wait. If your blood glucose levels are abnormal, it will be doing harm to you and your unborn child if you don't bring them back to normal.

Since your gestational diabetes will end when your pregnancy ends, your need to take insulin injections will cease when labor begins. Even when labor is induced, insulin injections usually are stopped before the process is started.

Diabetes Pills Aren't for You

No doubt you've heard that some people with diabetes take a pill—an antidiabetes pill—to control their blood glucose levels. That's true: Many people with type II, or noninsulin-dependent diabetes, can maintain good control by taking an oral medication. Unfortunately, women with gestational diabetes can't take any of the oral antidiabetes agents without causing potential harm to the unborn baby. These medications cross the placenta and can stimulate the insulin production by the beta cells in the pancreas of the fetus. Excess production of insulin can cause serious problems for your baby.

Some Basic Insulin Questions (and the Answers)

- *What is insulin?* Insulin is a hormone normally produced by the beta cells in the pancreas (a gland). Insulin works to take glucose out of the bloodstream into the cells of tissues, where the glucose is then "burned" as fuel.

- *Why does insulin need to be injected?* Since insulin is a protein, the digestive tract of the body cannot distinguish it from any other protein and will digest it and destroy its effectiveness if it is swallowed as an oral medication.

- *What is human insulin?* Human insulin is a synthetic insulin that is identical to the insulin produced in the human body. Before scientists developed the technique to produce human insulin, they relied on insulin obtained from the pancreas of slaughtered pigs and cows. Although pork and beef insulin worked to control blood glucose levels in humans, both of these products carried some risk of unwanted side effects, such as resistance and allergic reactions.

• *Are there any alternatives to injecting insulin?* Scientists have developed insulin that can be delivered by a nasal spray, as well as encapsulated insulin that can be swallowed but won't be destroyed by digestive juices. These forms, however, are still experimental and have not yet been approved for use by the Food & Drug Administration.

• *Are devices available that will either allow me to inject insulin without a needle or ease the injection process?* Yes, if needles make you uncomfortable, you may be interested in using a spray injector. This device uses air pressure to spray the correct dosage of insulin through the surface of your skin.

Another alternative may be using one of the assistive devices for insulin delivery, such as a pen-like device that automatically injects the correct dosage of insulin. Talk to your health care professional if you are interested in either of these methods of administering insulin.

Some people with diabetes use an insulin infusion pump to administer a continuous flow of insulin, supplemented by insulin injections at mealtimes. But for the type of insulin injection schedule that you will have to follow for the next few months, a pump is really not needed.

Understanding

Insulin Reactions

Sometimes people who must take insulin have a problem called "hypoglycemia" or low blood glucose. Most women with gestational diabetes won't have this problems, but it helps to know what it is and why it occurs on the off chance you may have some symptoms.

Hypoglycemia, which is also called an insulin reaction, usually occurs when the food you eat, the exercise you do, and the insulin you inject get out of balance. Insulin and exercise lower blood glucose, but food raises it. If you take too large a dose of insulin and exercise more than expected without eating enough, your blood glucose levels can plummet.

Checking your blood glucose is the most important thing you need to do if you are concerned that your blood glucose is low. There are also some symptoms, however. These include:

—Dizziness or shakiness

—Sweating

—Fast heart beat

—Clumsy or jerky movements

—Hunger

—Headache

—Mood swings or behavior changes, such as crying for no reason

—Pale skin

—Confusion or inability to concentrate

—Tingling sensations around the mouth

If you feel any of these warning signs, check your blood glucose level. If the level low, you need to eat or drink some form of sugar right away. Some examples are 3 or 4 pieces of hard candy or sugar cubes, 2 tablespoons of raisins, half a cup of orange juice, or an 8-ounce glass of milk. Check with your dietitian about what would work best for you.

After you have eaten something, wait 15 minutes, then check your blood again. If it is still low, eat some more of the sugars mentioned above or whatever your dietitian has recommended for you. After another 15 minutes, check your blood glucose again. If it is still low, call your health care provider for advice on what to do next.

Because of the risks of low blood glucose for insulin users, always carry some form of sugar with you when you exercise, travel, or even when you're at work. Unusual stress can cause blood glucose levels to drop suddenly, and it's best to be prepared.

Important note for insulin users:

Everyone who uses insulin should wear a medical identification bracelet or necklace or carry a card that says he or she uses insulin. If you were to have a serious reaction without recognizing the symptoms early, you could faint, and people around you might not know you were having an insulin reaction. This is another important reason for letting co-workers and friends and family all know about your gestational diabetes.

M o n i t o r i n g

How am I doing? That's a question you probably will want to ask yourself every morning. And it's a question your health care professional will ask you each time you visit, or call with a problem or question.

Where do you find the answer to this question? You can't just look in a mirror and get an accurate picture of what is going on inside of your body (although you can see general signs of good health or bad health). But you can get the correct—and timely—answer to this question by monitoring your own blood glucose.

Think about it. You can get the answer to the question, "How well am I doing with my weight?" by stepping on a bathroom scale and checking the numbers. That's a simple but basic technique of monitoring your weight.

You can also use a thermometer to monitor your body temperature to determine if you have a fever. That's another simple but basic method of monitoring one of the functions of your body.

Now it gets a bit more complex. To determine just how well you are doing with your gestational diabetes management program, you need to monitor your blood glucose. If your blood glucose measurement shows you are in the normal range, that's a sign that you are doing quite well. If your blood glucose measurement shows you are either above or below your normal range, it's a sign that things are not so good and you need to take some actions to fine-tune your management program to return your blood glucose levels to the normal range. Although a single above- or below-normal measurement is no cause for alarm, a pattern of repeated highs or lows raises a red flag that you should heed.

Fortunately for you, blood glucose monitoring is now relatively simple to do—although you need to spend time to learn how to do it right, and you need to spend money to purchase a blood glucose meter and the necessary supplies. We say you are fortunate because 15 years ago, you would not have been able to self-monitor your blood glucose. The equipment and the techniques started to come into general use only after 1980.

Self-monitoring of blood glucose provides you with a wealth of specific information.

- You can see what your blood glucose levels are at the exact time you do the measurement.

- You can see the effect a certain type amount of food has on your blood glucose levels.

- You can see the effect medication (particularly an insulin injection) has on your blood glucose levels.

- You can see the effect an exercise session has on your blood glucose levels.

- You can see the effect stress, illness, or lack of sleep has on your blood glucose levels.

- You can see, precisely, if the ill feelings you are having (headache, fatigue, and so on) are symptoms of a high or a low blood glucose level, or whether they have other causes.

- You can see, in general terms, just how well all of the parts of your diabetes management plan are fitting together to ensure your good health and the health of your baby.

The most important thing you can do during the next few months—until you deliver your child—is to keep your blood glucose levels within a normal range. Self-monitoring of blood glucose will tell you whether you are achieving this goal.

Your basic goal is to keep your fasting blood glucose between 60 to 80 mg/dl (3.3 to 4.4 mmol/L) and your one-hour post-meal blood glucose levels under 120 mg/dl (6.7 mmol/L). For pregnant women who do not have gestational diabetes, blood glucose levels rarely exceed 100 mg/dl (5.6 mmol/L) and range from 60 to 80 mg/dl (3.3 to 4.4 mmol/L) fasting and 120 mg/dl (6.7 mmol/L) one hour after eating.

Here are some of the things that can affect your blood glucose levels or show up in your blood glucose measurements:

- the quantity of foods you eat

- the kinds of foods you eat

- quantity of simple sugars in the food you eat

- what time you eat a meal or snack

- time since you last ate

- type of exercise

- intensity of exercise

- length of time you exercise

- stress, such as from an argument with your spouse

- a cold or other minor illness

- an upset stomach

- diarrhea

- nausea

- anxiety about your pregnancy

- anger about having diabetes

- your insulin dosage

- timing of your insulin injection

- the type of insulin you inject

- the technique you use to inject insulin

- your technique for measuring your blood glucose

- the condition of your blood glucose test strips

- the condition and cleanliness of your blood glucose monitor

- the reaction of your body, and that of your baby, to every-thing in your life

With so many factors affecting blood glucose levels, it's easy to see just how important blood glucose monitoring is.

Learning to measure your blood glucose levels is fairly quick and easy. Your health care professional can explain the process and teach you how to do it properly. It will take some practice on your part, but the time you spend in learning to do it right will be worth it.

Your health care professional will discuss with you the various choices you have in blood glucose meters; many different types are available, at different prices, and with different benefits. Once you have selected a meter, you will need to learn how to use it properly. Most meter packages include a tutorial (audio- or videotape), but hands-on instruction from a health professional will make learning easier.

Although procedures vary with the different meters, the basic techniques follow a pattern:

- You stick your fingertip with a lancet, or use a spring-loaded device that does this for you.

- You place a drop of blood from the fingertip puncture on a chemically treated pad or strip.

- This strip or pad is placed in the blood glucose meter and an electronic brain within the meter "reads" the reaction between the chemicals in the test strip or pad and the glucose in your blood. The more glucose, the greater the reaction. The meter converts the reaction results into a blood glucose level (in mg/dl) and displays the result on a screen. All of this takes place within seconds after you start the procedure.

When you see the numbers on the screen, you can do a number of things.

- If the numbers are within the normal range, you can log the results in your record book and give yourself a pat on the back for a job well done.

- If the numbers are slightly above or below your normal range, you can log the numbers in your record book and keep a lookout for patterns of above- or below-normal measurements. For example, if your log shows that you consistently run above normal after you eat lunch, that's a signal for you to do one or more of the following things:

  —cut down on the total amount of food you eat

  —decrease the amount of carbohydrates in your meal

  —increase your physical activity after lunch

  —adjust the amount of insulin you inject before lunch.

Before you adjust anything, however, get instructions from your health care professional on what adjustments you should make and when you should make them (all based on specific blood glucose measurements).

- If the numbers are significantly above or below normal, you need to take immediate action. For example, if you inject insulin and one hour later you get a blood glucose measurement below 60 mg/dl (3.3 mmol/L), you need to drink a cup of milk or eat a serving of fruit or juice to prevent a low blood glucose attack. Then get advice on how to decrease your dose of insulin so this problem will not recur.

When and How Often Should You Measure Your Blood Glucose?

The answer to this questions is quite simple—**as often as possible.** The more monitoring you do, the more precisely you will be able to take control and maintain control of your diabetes.

Your health care professional will work with you to design a monitoring schedule especially for you. The frequency of monitoring will be based on the severity of your gestational diabetes, your health history and health status, the stage and progress of your pregnancy, and last, but not least, your willingness to participate in an intensive treatment program to improve your health and the health of your unborn child.

If you manage your gestational diabetes with diet and exercise alone, you will measure your blood glucose four times a day. You will do a measurement when you wake up in the morning, and one hour after each meal.

If you manage your gestational diabetes with insulin injections, plus diet and exercise, your blood glucose monitoring schedule will be more complicated. You need to perform eight blood glucose measurements each day—one hour before and one hour after each meal, before you go to sleep and in the middle of the night at about 3 a.m.

In addition to the regularly scheduled measurements, you may be asked to (or want to) measure your blood glucose before and after you exercise, and when you are feeling under the weather.

Record Keeping

Don't rely on your memory to keep track of your blood glucose measurements The specific numbers and the dates and times you did the measurements are very important. Some blood glucose meters do have built-in memories to record blood glucose measurements (including date and time). If yours does, that's good; but you'll also want to keep a record of food, exercise, insulin (and other medications), special events, illnesses, and so on. To do this effectively, you will want to keep a diabetes record book. A sample record is included on pages 112 through 125.

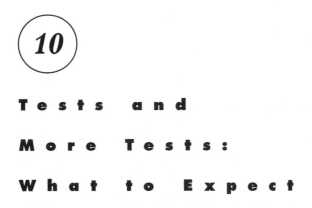

Tests and More Tests: What to Expect

In addition to blood glucose monitoring, there are other types of tests and measurements you need to be aware of. Many women with gestational diabetes are asked to do a routine fasting urine ketone test. You may be spilling ketones into your urine if your intake of carbohydrates is too low, if you are following a meal plan that is too low in calories, or if you skip a meal (or snack) or two.

Ketones are formed when your body starts to burn fat stores for energy because there is not enough insulin available to work on the glucose in your blood or when you radically reduce the glucose available by following a starvation or fasting diet—which is a strong no-no for pregnant women.

The ketone test uses a simple dip-and-read strip that you place in a urine sample or your urine stream. If you are spilling ketones into your urine, the strip changes color. These test strips can also indicate the amount of ketones present. Large amounts of ketones in your urine may be a danger signal, and you should notify your health care professional immediately.

If your blood glucose measurement shows that your glucose level is 240 mg/dl (13.3 mmol/L) or higher, then you certainly should do a urine ketone test. You can easily learn how to test your urine for ketones and can keep the testing supplies at home for use when needed.

The other types of tests and measurements are done in your doctor's office. One of these tests is called a glycosylated hemoglobin assay (or hemoglobin A_1C test). This procedure measures the amount of hemoglobin (red blood cells) that have been linked with glucose in your bloodstream. A lab technician or nurse will take a sample of your blood from a vein. Results are usually available within a half hour, thanks to new table-top instruments that can be used in the doctor's office laboratory.

The result of the glycosylated hemoglobin assay shows the average level of blood glucose in your body during the past six weeks. This is different from the blood glucose measurement you do at home, which shows the blood glucose level at the time of the measurement.

Your doctor may do a glycosylated hemoglobin assay at the time your gestational diabetes is diagnosed (to see what happened with your blood glucose before the diagnosis) and may do another one about six weeks later (to see how the program has been working). Ideally, hemoglobin A_1C should be measured every month to double-check the blood glucose monitoring. After you give birth, your doctor may recommend you have this test every six months or annually to make sure you are doing well and check for warning signs of type II, noninsulin-dependent diabetes.

In addition to diabetes-related tests and measurements, your doctor may perform the following to monitor the health and development of your unborn child.

- Ultrasound, alpha-fetoprotein and genetic testing, if it has not been done earlier in your pregnancy

- Fetal activity determination

- Biophysical fetal testing, such as weekly or semiweekly non-stress tests, contraction stress tests, or biophysical profiles

- Fetal lung-maturity analysis (through amniocentesis) if elective delivery is planned

Here are brief descriptions of some of these tests.

Ultrasound. This procedure uses short pulses of high-frequency, low-intensity sound waves to safely provide a "picture" of the placenta, your uterus, and the baby growing within it. Through ultrasound, your doctor can accurately determine the growth and development of the fetus, and the due date. A precise due date may be quite important if your doctor must induce your labor or perform a cesarean delivery. The ultrasound procedure does not expose you or your baby to radiation. The procedure also can be used to guide the doctor if he or she is performing amniocentesis (see page 82).

Fetal movement measurements (performed by you but reported to your doctor). During your last trimester, your doctor may ask you to count the number of times the baby moves or kicks during a two-hour period. Three or more movements during this time is considered normal. If you count less, or significantly more movements, that's your signal to contact your doctor.

Amniocentesis. For this procedure, the doctor removes a small amount of fluid from the amniotic sac sometime during mid-pregnancy. By analyzing this fluid, genetic abnormalities, such as Down syndrome, in the fetus may be detected. The procedure, done late in pregnancy, can determine if the baby's lungs are mature enough to withstand early delivery.

Nonstress tests. Electronic monitors are held in place over your abdomen with an elasticized belt. The monitors detect contractions of your uterus—contractions you may or may not be able to feel—while you lie at rest. You will also be given a pen to draw a line on the computer printout each time you feel your baby move. Each time the baby moves, his or her heart rate should go up at least by 15 beats per minute. Lack of rise of the baby's pulse rate with movement may mean the baby is sick. A biophysical profile may then be performed, which is a detailed exam of the baby using ultrasonography.

Blood pressure and weight. At each office visit, your doctor will also measure your blood pressure (you may be at increased risk for hypertension) and your weight (control of weight within set parameters is a must).

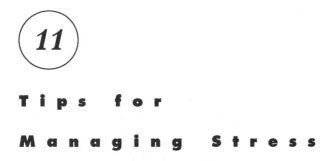

Tips for Managing Stress

Stress is a normal part of every pregnancy. Your body is changing, you have new demands—physically and mentally, you have concerns about your baby, and you are thinking about how your life will change in the future. Gestational diabetes carries many additional stresses. You need to eat right and on schedule, you need to take time to exercise, you need to monitor your blood glucose, and perhaps you need to use insulin.

With all these stresses, some guidelines for stress management can be very helpful as you cope from day to day.

- *Listen to your body.* Tune in to the signals that tell you you are feeling stress. Are your neck muscles tight, does you head ache, do you have butterflies in your stomach? These are all important signals. Listen to them and zero in on what you might do to change the situation.

- *Look at your life realistically.* Take a step back and look at the demands that are causing your stress. What can you do to eliminate them? Are there just too many demands? Can someone help you meet some of them? Learn to ask for help and to say no when you feel you can't handle more stress or responsibility.

- *Become alert to ways you cause stress for yourself.* Are you expecting too much of yourself? This is not the time to prove you are a superwoman. Self-imposed deadlines, critical self-talk, and overly high expectations can be changed. Don't become trapped by your own unrealistic goals for yourself.

- *Make good choices.* Be kind and positive with yourself. Tell yourself what a good job you're doing—and say it often and with conviction. If your goals are unrealistic, change them. Chances are they're your internal goals and no one else will even notice.

- *Learn to relax.* Buy yourself a relaxation tape, listen to soothing music, take a bubble bath, or imagine yourself in a quiet, peaceful setting and just enjoy the comfort for a few minutes. If you can't make these work for you, ask your health care professional for advice on muscle relaxation techniques or classes for learning how to relax.

- *Enlist support.* Let your friends, family, and especially your partner help you. Tell them what you need and what they can do to ease the burdens you're feeling. And don't forget to talk with your health care providers. They can give good information and help you face the challenges you meet.

- *Take time for regular exercise.* This is a great stress reducer. Walking is a perfect way to enjoy the calm and wonder of nature and to work off some of that worry.

- *Use your sense of humor.* Laughter is a wonderful stress reliever. If you can't think of anything to laugh about, just stand in front of a mirror and force yourself to laugh. Soon you begin to enjoy the humor of your own laughter. This is a great skill to maintain throughout your child-rearing years, as well.

- *Be an active partner in your own health care.* Get all the information you need to feel you are in control of your pregnancy and your diabetes. Ask lots of questions and learn everything you can about what's happening to your body.

- *Take good care of yourself.* Don't short-change yourself on what you need to stay well, whether it's a good night's sleep, some time for yourself, some help with the housework, or a day off from work. Put yourself and your health right up there at the top of the list for the next few months. It's the best investment you can make right now.

12

What to Expect on Birth Day

It's the big day for Kate. She's sure (this time) that she really is in labor. Her mind is filled with questions: Should she wake up Dave now (in the middle of the night) or wait a little longer? Did she pack her favorite robe? Has she remembered everything on her checklist? Has she remembered everything her health care team has instructed her to do when the big day arrives?

Fortunately, before the big day, Kate wrote down all the instructions her health care team gave her, showed the list to her husband, and even posted a note on the coffee machine to remind Dave where the instruction list was. She even wrote down the 24-hour phone number of her health care team.

What a relief. When she reminded herself that she had followed all the proper procedures she was able to calm down. She felt confident everything was ready.

When the contractions became stronger and more regular, she knew it was time to wake Dave.

He jumped out of bed with a scared, confused look on his face. "What do you want me to do first, honey?"

Luckily, Kate already had her panic attack, so she could calm him down, tell him to get the checklist and suitcase, and start the car.

Without hesitation, Dave did what she asked. The two went safely and quickly to the hospital in plenty of time for the birth of their first child— a beautiful, healthy baby girl named Jackie.

The start of labor is the moment you've been waiting for all of these past nine months, and especially during the last four or so months, since you were diagnosed as having gestational diabetes.

You'll be pleased to know that most women with gestational diabetes can complete pregnancy and begin the labor process naturally. Some, however, may require an elective delivery, with labor induced by a medication called oxytocin. And some women may need a cesarean section because the baby is too large or in distress or because the woman's body may not be able to handle a vaginal birth.

A "birthing" class, such as one for natural childbirth, can help prepare for this dramatic event. But you will also need to maintain good control of your blood glucose levels right up to the time you enter the hospital to deliver your baby.

In-hospital delivery, rather than home birthing, is highly recommended for women who have gestational diabetes. The hospital and its professional staff will be prepared to handle any problems that may occur during the labor and delivery process.

If your blood glucose levels are elevated or become elevated during labor, your baby's blood glucose levels will also rise above normal. Immediately after birth, the baby's blood glucose may drop to a dangerously low level (hypoglycemia) as the result of the baby's high insulin levels, which are normal right after birth.

If you have not needed insulin as part of your gestational diabetes management plan, then you will not need to take insulin injections during labor or delivery. Even those women who have needed insulin during pregnancy usually need no more insulin once the contractions begin. Labor is a form of exercise, and the exercise "burns" the sugar and thus insulin may not be necessary.

Once you give birth, your need for insulin injections stops (for most women with gestational diabetes). Your blood glucose levels will return to normal and, with a little effort on your part, can stay that way.

When you deliver the placenta (afterbirth), you will also remove the source of the extra hormones that created the insulin resistance that led to your development of gestational diabetes. Unlike people who have the other kinds of diabetes (type I, insulin-dependent, and type II, noninsulin-dependent) which are present for a lifetime, gestational diabetes disappears when you give birth. And, you can be assured that your baby will not be born with diabetes.

However, both you and your baby are at risk for developing type II diabetes later in life, and you need to take steps to lower these risks. You are also at extremely high risks for developing gestational diabetes if you become pregnant again. Before we explain how to lower diabetes risks for you and your baby, you need to be aware of some other health concerns for your newborn.

If your blood glucose levels were elevated during the 24 hours before delivery, there is a chance that your baby may be at risk for post-birth low blood glucose levels (hypoglycemia). Blood glucose measurements will provide accurate information on both you and your newborn. If your baby's blood glucose levels are too low, he or she can be given extra glucose to bring the levels into the normal range.

As we discussed earlier, another problem that can develop in the newborn of a mother with gestational diabetes is jaundice. To briefly review, jaundice occurs when a substance called bilirubin is released after extra blood cells in the baby's system are destroyed (for reasons unrelated to your gestational diabetes). Bilirubin contains a pigment that causes a yellow discoloration of the skin. A minor degree of jaundice is common in many newborns.

The condition is treated by placing the baby under special lights that help the body absorb and excrete the bilirubin and eliminate the yellow pigmentation. In severe cases, which are quite rare, a blood transfusion may be needed.

If you have followed your prescribed management program to control your gestational diabetes, you have greatly reduced the risk that your baby will be born with birth defects or other health problems related to your body's problems in handling glucose.

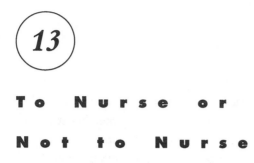

13

To Nurse or Not to Nurse

One way to start your newborn on a proper nutritional path is to breast-feed. Nearly all women can breast-feed, and most find it emotionally satisfying. It helps you bond with your baby, it's inexpensive, and it's convenient.

Another plus for breast-feeding is the fact that breast milk contains antibodies that fight certain infections. You're helping protect your baby's health and you're helping him or her grow and feel secure.

Breast-feeding also can help you lose weight—both weight you gained during pregnancy and weight you may have carried before you became pregnant.

A word of caution about breast-feeding and *weight loss*. Most women will lose between 12 and 15 pounds during the first week after delivery. After that, the weight you gained during pregnancy should come off gradually, over about a three-month period.

If your doctor recommends that you lose weight, it's all right to begin while you are breast-feeding. However, it probably is best to wait two to four weeks after your baby is born before you start a weight loss plan.

Be sure you ask for guidance as you lose weight. Remember that a gradual loss is the safest approach. Also, weight lost slowly is much more likely to stay lost. Don't try any fad diets or quick-loss plans while you're nursing your baby. Also, remember it is very important to maintain your intake of calcium, vitamins, and water so you don't jeopardize your own or your infant's good health.

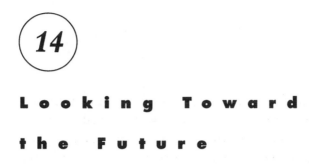

14

Looking Toward the Future

Since both you and your newborn baby are at increased risk for developing diabetes, you'll want to make some immediate plans to reduce these risks.

You are a double risk: You have over a 70 percent chance of developing gestational diabetes if you become pregnant again, and you have an increased risk of developing type II diabetes sometime in the not-so-distant future. In a clinical study, scientists found that more than 50 percent of women who had gestational diabetes develop type II diabetes within 15 years after the pregnancy.

But in addition to having had gestational diabetes, other risk factors also play a role in your chances of developing type II diabetes. Some of these risk factors are under your control and some are not.

For instance, you can't change risk factors such as your age and your family history. Type II diabetes develops more often in people who are over 40 years and in people who have blood relatives who have type II diabetes. But you can change another risk factor. Type II diabetes develops more often in people who are overweight.

As we said earlier, most women lose between 12 and 15 pounds during the first week after they give birth. An within about 3 months after your baby's birth, you should lose all the weight you gained during pregnancy. You often can do this by just following a regular diet and by doing the routine activities of caring for a newborn.

But if you carried too many pounds before you became pregnant, or if you gained too much weight during pregnancy, you need to take action to lose those extra pounds and keep them off.

Forget about quick weight-loss diets and miracle diet pills. They don't work in the long run. It may do your body more harm if you lose extra weight through these programs than if you don't lose the weight at all! Also, the weight is likely to come back quickly when it's lost quickly.

The answer, which is quite simplified here, is to change your eating habits and lifestyle. Most people who are overweight get this way because they eat too much food, eat the wrong kinds of foods, or don't get enough physical activity. They live to eat rather than eat to live.

To get on the right nutrition track, talk to the dietitian who developed the meal plan you followed to help control your gestational diabetes. The dietitian will be able to analyze your eating habits and preferences and then recommend an eating program (not a diet) that you, your spouse, and eventually, your newborn child can follow. The program will be built on a healthy meal plan that is nutritious and tasty, too.

When you follow a healthy eating program in your household, your baby will grow up expecting the right kinds and amounts of nutritious foods (rather than the fast foods and sugary snacks the youngster sees on television).

As the mother, you are a role model for your child. If you follow healthy eating habits, your child will follow your lead. If you are able to instill these good eating habits in your child, his or her chances of being overweight and developing type II diabetes as an adult are greatly reduced.

Although your lifestyle for the first few months after birth will be seriously disrupted by the baby, and your physical activities will be increased (along with a decrease in sleep and rest), you cannot neglect regular exercise.

As soon as possible after you give birth (within 3 to 4 weeks after normal birth, 6 to 8 weeks after cesarean delivery) you need to return to your regular exercise program. Exercise will tone up your muscles (getting rid of the flabby and stretched skin), and increase your flexibility, energy (really), and physical endurance. Exercise can also help you to lose weight when you follow a prescribed reduced-calorie diet. It can also help keep your blood glucose levels in good control and reduce your future risks for heart and circulatory system disease.

If you were an avid runner, tennis player, jogger, or biker before you became pregnant, you can go back to these favorite exercises. The restrictions placed on you concerning exercise choices during pregnancy are lifted after you have given birth.

If, however, you were a couch potato before you got pregnant, you may need some advice and counseling on exercise choices and techniques before starting a new program. Talk to your doctor or another member of your health care team about starting an exercise program. A team member may be able to give you advice or refer you to an exercise expert at the local hospital, community center, or health club.

If you are new to exercise, remember that you need to start small and build gradually. Pick an activity or two that you like (such as biking, walking, or swimming) and then set aside time to do it on a regular basis. Meeting the demands of caring for a baby—and the rest of your family—may make you feel there are not enough hours in the day to allot some to exercise. You'll need help and cooperation from other family members to allow you time for exercise.

To be effective, your exercise should be of moderate intensity (brisk walking, for instance), should last about 30 minutes (plus a 10-minute warm-up and 10-minute cool-down period) and should be done every other day.

Glucose Monitoring

Don't throw away your blood glucose meter and strips after you give birth. You will need this equipment to check on your blood glucose levels on a regular basis. You'll find that doing blood glucose measurements when you are on a weight-loss diet can be very educational, showing how certain foods, kinds, and quantities affect your blood glucose levels.

Monitoring of your blood glucose levels can also help you detect any developing problems with the way your body handles the glucose from the food you eat. It can provide you and your doctor an early warning sign that type II diabetes may be developing.

In addition to your at-home glucose monitoring, your doctor will also recommend that you visit the office within 3 months after birth to take an oral glucose-tolerance test—the same test you took when the diagnosis of gestational diabetes was made, although this drink is smaller (75 gm. after birth compared with 100 gm. during pregnancy). After the 3-month checkup, you should also get this test once a year.

If the test shows that you are developing (and this doesn't happen very often) type II diabetes, you can start on a management program immediately (usually using diet and exercise alone). Even though newly diagnosed type II diabetes may not have many distressing symptoms, the sooner you are able to control and normalize your blood glucose levels, the better able you will be to avoid, postpone, or reduce the severity of potential diabetes complications, including heart disease and circulatory system disorders.

If you are planning to become pregnant again, you need to start a special program before your conceive. This program should be designed to enable you to lose excess weight before you become pregnant and to keep your blood glucose levels within the normal range.

Birth Control

As part of your planning for the future, you should consider birth control—whether or not you want to have another child. A number of birth control options are available to you. The option you choose should be one that fits within your lifestyle, is acceptable to you and your partner, and has a high success rate and a low amount of health risk.

Here are some of the birth control methods available today:

Oral contraceptives (the pill). Oral contraceptives are 99 percent effective when used according to directions. The pill is one of the most popular methods of birth control in use today. Although effective, it carries a risk of side effects. The pill may not be for you if you have a medical history of heart disease, stroke, high blood pressure, or blood vessel problems (such as phlebitis). Your health risks are increased if you use the pill and smoke or are over the age of 30. Oral contraceptives come in many dosage forms and combinations and require a doctor's prescription. The low dose pills do not cause your diabetes to come back. If your diabetes does come back and you are not pregnant again, it would have happened even if you did not start the pill. Check with your doctor concerning whether you are a candidate for an oral contraceptive and, if so, which kind is best for you.

Injection/Implant. The hormones contained in oral contraceptives can also be injected or implanted to provide long-term birth control. The injected form works for about 3 months. Implants provide protection for up to 5 years. The implant, however, can be removed during this time if you desire to become pregnant again. The hormone in these injections or implant is a high enough dose that it may bring back your diabetes. Therefore, these usually are not first-choice contraceptives for women with previous gestational diabetes.

Diaphragm. When fitted properly and used correctly, the diaphragm can be up to 95 percent effective. Although there are no side effects with its use, the diaphragm requires advance planning for proper insertion before intercourse. It may be used in conjunction with spermicidal jelly or foam to increase its effectiveness. The diaphragm must be fitted by a health care professional, who will also instruct you on how to use it properly.

Condom. When used properly, a condom may be an effective method of birth control (up to 85 percent effective), particularly when combined with a spermicidal jelly or foam. Condoms are also effective barriers to the spread of sexually transmitted disease. Condom use requires active cooperation from the male partner. (A female-use condom has recently been developed and marketed, but it has not been available long enough to develop statistics on its effectiveness.)

The sponge. This is a sponge-like object that contains a spermicidal gel and is placed in the vagina prior to intercourse. The reliability of sponge has not yet been proven.

Intrauterine device (IUD). Because the IUD was suspected of causing pelvic infections, many manufacturers stopped producing and selling these devices. The IUDs were found to be highly effective, but carried some health risks. Check with your doctor concerning the availability and suitability of an IUD if you are interested in using this method.

Rhythm and withdrawal. These two methods of birth control are the least effective techniques. The rhythm relies on restricting intercourse to only certain times during the woman's menstrual cycle when she is least likely to be fertile. This method, however, is not recommended for women who have a history of gestational diabetes.

The withdrawal method (withdrawing the penis from the vagina before ejaculation occurs) requires precise timing. Because of this, it is rarely effective as a birth control method for anyone.

Sterilization. If you do not plan to have any more children, you or your spouse can consider a permanent method of birth control.

For men, the technique is called a vasectomy (a surgical procedure to prevent sperm from being ejaculated). Vasectomies can be performed in a doctor's office under local anesthesia. There is also a procedure to reverse a vasectomy, restoring function, but the results are mixed.

For women, the sterilization technique is called a tubal ligation. The fallopian tubes through which the eggs (ova) pass on the way to the uterus are blocked or cut. This procedure is generally done under general anesthesia, often in a 1-day surgery center. Once it is done, it rarely can be undone.

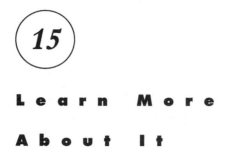

Learn More About It

Many resources are available to help you learn more about diabetes and diabetes management. A first stop might be the local office of the American Diabetes Association (listed in your telephone directory). Many ADA units conduct educational courses for people with diabetes. Some ADA units also sponsor support groups for people who share similar interests or problems, such as gestational diabetes. Most ADA offices also have lists of books, as well as educational booklets, free or at a minimal cost.

The following publications are highly recommended, particularly for helping in meal planning.

Exchange Lists for Meal Planning, Family Cookbook. and *Holiday Cookbook.* Contact ADA, 1-800-232-3472 for ordering information.

Fast Food Facts, Exchanges for All Occasions (revised edition), and *The Joy of Snacks.* Available from CHRONIMED, Inc., (see telephone numbers listed below for information on ordering).

For basic diabetes education, you may consider these publications available from CHRONIMED:

Learning to Live Well with Diabetes and *A Touch of Diabetes.* Contact CHRONIMED for information about ordering by calling (outside Minnesota) 1-800-848-2793; (inside Minnesota) 612-546-1146.

Glossary of Terms

On the following pages is a glossary of some of the terms we have used in this book, along with a simplified definition of the terms. If our explanation is not sufficiently detailed for you, we recommend that you ask your diabetes care professional for an expanded definition (in language you can understand).

Amniocentesis: One of the procedures that may be done during pregnancy to determine if the developing fetus is carrying certain genetic defects. The procedure also can determine the sex of the fetus.

Biophysical profile: A procedure that may be done during pregnancy to evaluate fetal movement, muscle tone, lung development, and the amount of amniotic fluid in the amniotic sac (the "water bag" in which the fetus develops).

Carbohydrates: One of the three basic nutrients (along with protein and fat) that supply calories to the body. Carbohydrates include sugars and starches, and are most commonly present in nonanimal foods (such as plants). Carbohydrates are classified as simple (such as table sugar) or complex (such as vegetables and grains).

Diabetes (mellitus): A group of disorders that involve the inability of the person's body to properly use glucose (derived from food). This results in a buildup of glucose in the bloodstream, and the spilling of glucose into the urine. There are various forms of diabetes mellitus. The most common ones are: type I, insulin-dependent; type II, noninsulin-dependent; and gestational diabetes.

Fat: Another of the three basic nutrients. Fats are commonly present in animal food sources, but are also found in nuts (coconuts) and some plants (palm, olive). There are three major forms of fat: saturated (from animals), monounsaturated (from olives), and polyunsaturated (from corn). Although fat is an essential nutrient, most Americans ingest too much fat, and this excess fat is deposited in the body's arteries, where it may eventually cause heart attacks and stroke.

Glucose: The basic form of sugar used by the body's cells for energy. All digestible food is changed into glucose within the body. Simple sugar (table sugar) is converted to glucose the fastest; proteins are converted to glucose more slowly, and fats are converted much more slowly.

Glucose-tolerance test: This is the diagnostic procedure used to confirm whether a person has gestational diabetes (or other forms of diabetes). During this procedure, the person ingests a liquid containing 100 grams of glucose, and then has consecutive blood glucose measurements taken each hour for 3 hours. The information from these measurements provides the doctor with a picture of how the person's body metabolizes the precise glucose amount contained in the special glucose drink. This test usually is given to pregnant women after a glucose screening test indicates there may be some problems. The screening test should be conducted between the 24th and 28th week of pregnancy.

Hyperglycemia: A term used to describe the situation when blood glucose levels are above the normal range. Prolonged high or extremely high glucose levels can lead to serious and sometimes life-threatening diabetes complications, for both the mother with gestational diabetes and for the developing fetus.

Hypoglycemia: A term used to describe the situation when blood glucose levels are below the normal range. When blood glucose levels drop below normal, the person may develop dramatic symptoms (irritability, irrational behavior, headaches, dizziness, and so on). If left untreated, hypoglycemia may lead to unconsciousness and even coma.

Insulin: This is a hormone secreted by the beta cells located in the pancreas. Insulin's major function is to enable glucose (derived from foods, and carried in the bloodstream) to enter the body's cells, where it is burned as "fuel." In all forms of diabetes, the function of insulin is disturbed; either the body develops "resistance" to the action of naturally secreted insulin, or the body does not produce enough insulin, or the body does not produce any insulin. Some people with diabetes require injections to allow glucose to move from the bloodstream into the cells. Without enough functioning insulin available, unused glucose piles up in the bloodstream and, eventually, this extra glucose severely damages nerves, blood vessels, and other organs within the body.

Insulin resistance: This is a condition in which insulin produced in the body, or injected, is blocked from doing its job. This blocking may be caused by excess hormones produced by the placenta. Such hormone production increases gradually throughout pregnancy but peaks in the last trimester. Insulin resistance is also linked to excess weight. Fat cells in the body can block the "receptors" on cells and thus block the insulin's access to the cells.

Ketones: These are chemicals produced when the body burns stored fat for energy. Excess ketones are spilled into the urine, where they can be detected with a simple test. Ketones may appear in the urine when blood glucose levels are far above normal, or when there is not enough carbohydrate available to convert into glucose (such as when a person is fasting, or just not eating enough carbohydrates).

Macrosomia: This is a scientific term used to describe a condition when the developing fetus or newborn baby is considerably larger than normal. This is a preventable complication of gestational diabetes; tight control of blood glucose levels can greatly reduce the health risks for both the mother and the baby.

Nutrients: This is a term used to describe the substances found in foods and needed by the body to support organ function. Nutrients include proteins, carbohydrates, fats, vitamins, and minerals. A "proper" balance of nutrients is required to maintain a healthy life.

Placenta: The organ that connects the fetus to the mother's uterus. The placenta obtains nutrients from the mother's bloodstream and transports these nutrients across the umbilical cord to the developing fetus. The placenta secretes hormones that are necessary for the proper growth and development of the fetus and eventually for the process of labor and delivery. Placental hormones can also increase the mother's resistance to the insulin her cells produce.

Protein: Another essential nutrient, usually found in animal-source foods, but also present in nuts, seeds, legumes (beans and peas), and whole grains.

Trimester: One third of the pregnancy, which normally runs 40 weeks. The first trimester includes weeks 1 to 12, the second includes weeks 13 to 26, and the third, weeks 27 to 40.

Biographical Information

Lois Jovanovic-Peterson, MD, is Senior Scientist at the Sansum Medical Research Foundation in Santa Barbara, California. She recently served as editor-in-chief of the book *Medical Management of Pregnancy Complicated by Diabetes*, which was published as part of the Clinical Education Series by the American Diabetes Association.

She has authored many scientific papers dealing with diabetes and pregnancy—including quite a few focused specifically on gestational diabetes.

Dr. Jovanovic-Peterson is coauthor (with Dr. Charles Peterson and Morton B. Stone) of the book *A Touch of Diabetes*, published by CHRONIMED, Inc., and coauthor (with June Biermann and Barbara Toohey) of *The Diabetic Woman*, published by Jeremy P. Tarcher, Inc.

Morton B. Stone is the editorial director of the magazine *Diabetes in the News*. He is coauthor of *A Touch of Diabetes* and has written many patient-education booklets for people with diabetes. He is an honorary member of the American Association of Diabetes Educators.

Sample Record Pages

Day	Time	Insulin Dose/Type	Blood Glucose Test				Urine Ketone Tests	Notes
			Breakfast	Lunch	Dinner	Bedtime		
			before / 1 hr. after	before / 1 hr. after	before / 1hr. after			

Food

Breakfast	CHO	Portion	Lunch	CHO	Portion	Dinner	CHO	Portion
Snack	CHO	Portion	Snack	CHO	Portion	Snack	CHO	Portion

Exercise

Type		Duration	

Comments

112

Day	Time	Insulin Dose/Type	Blood Glucose Test				Urine Ketone Tests	Notes
			Breakfast	**Lunch**	**Dinner**	**Bedtime**		
			before / 1 hr. after	before / 1 hr. after	before / 1hr. after			

Food

	CHO	Portion		CHO	Portion		CHO	Portion
Breakfast			Lunch			Dinner		
Snack			Snack			Snack		

Exercise

Type	Duration

Comments

Blood Glucose Test

Day	Time	Insulin Dose/Type	Breakfast before / 1 hr. after	Lunch before / 1 hr. after	Dinner before / 1hr. after	Bedtime	Urine Ketone Tests	Notes

Food

Breakfast	CHO	Portion	Lunch	CHO	Portion	Dinner	CHO	Portion
Snack	CHO	Portion	Snack	CHO	Portion	Snack	CHO	Portion

Exercise

Type	Duration

Comments

114

Day	Time	Insulin Dose/Type	Blood Glucose Test							Urine Ketone Tests	Notes
			Breakfast		Lunch		Dinner		Bedtime		
			before	1 hr. after	before	1 hr. after	before	1hr. after			

Food

Breakfast	CHO	Portion	Lunch	CHO	Portion	Dinner	CHO	Portion
Snack	CHO	Portion	Snack	CHO	Portion	Snack	CHO	Portion

Exercise

Type		Duration

Comments

115

			Blood Glucose Test							Urine Ketone Tests	Notes
Day	Time	Insulin Dose/Type	Breakfast		Lunch		Dinner		Bedtime		
			before	1 hr. after	before	1 hr. after	before	1 hr. after			

Food

Breakfast	CHO	Portion	Lunch	CHO	Portion	Dinner	CHO	Portion
Snack	CHO	Portion	Snack	CHO	Portion	Snack	CHO	Portion

Exercise

Type		Duration

Comments

Blood Glucose Test

Day	Time	Insulin Dose/Type	Breakfast		Lunch		Dinner		Bedtime	Urine Ketone Tests	Notes
			before	1 hr. after	before	1 hr. after	before	1 hr. after			

Food

Breakfast	CHO	Portion	Lunch	CHO	Portion	Dinner	CHO	Portion
Snack	CHO	Portion	Snack	CHO	Portion			

Exercise

Type	Duration

Comments

117

Day	Time	Insulin Dose/Type	Blood Glucose Test				Urine Ketone Tests	Notes
			Breakfast	Lunch	Dinner	Bedtime		
			before / 1 hr. after	before / 1 hr. after	before / 1hr. after			

Food

Breakfast	CHO	Portion	Lunch	CHO	Portion	Dinner	CHO	Portion
Snack	CHO	Portion	Snack	CHO	Portion	Snack	CHO	Portion

Exercise

Type	Duration

Comments

118

Blood Glucose Test

Day	Time	Insulin Dose/Type	Breakfast (before / 1 hr. after)	Lunch (before / 1 hr. after)	Dinner (before / 1 hr. after)	Bedtime	Urine Ketone Tests	Notes

Food

Breakfast	CHO	Portion	Lunch	CHO	Portion	Dinner	CHO	Portion

Snack	CHO	Portion	Snack	CHO	Portion

Exercise

Type	Duration

Comments

119

Day	Time	Insulin Dose/Type	Blood Glucose Test				Urine Ketone Tests	Notes
			Breakfast	Lunch	Dinner	Bedtime		
			before / 1 hr. after	before / 1 hr. after	before / 1 hr. after			

Food

Breakfast	CHO	Portion	Lunch	CHO	Portion	Dinner	CHO	Portion
Snack	CHO	Portion	Snack	CHO	Portion	Snack	CHO	Portion

Exercise

Type	Duration

Comments

Day	Time	Insulin Dose/Type	Blood Glucose Test							Urine Ketone Tests	Notes
			Breakfast		Lunch		Dinner		Bedtime		
			before	1 hr. after	before	1 hr. after	before	1 hr. after			

Food

Breakfast	CHO	Portion	Lunch	CHO	Portion	Dinner	CHO	Portion
Snack	CHO	Portion	Snack	CHO	Portion	Snack	CHO	Portion

Exercise

Type		Duration	

Comments

121

Blood Glucose Test

Day	Time	Insulin Dose/Type	Breakfast		Lunch		Dinner		Bedtime	Urine Ketone Tests	Notes
			before / 1 hr. after		before / 1 hr. after		before / 1hr. after				

Food

Breakfast	CHO	Portion	Lunch	CHO	Portion	Dinner	CHO	Portion
Snack	CHO	Portion	Snack	CHO	Portion			

Exercise

Type	Duration

Comments

Day	Time	Insulin Dose/Type	Blood Glucose Test				Urine Ketone Tests	Notes
			Breakfast	Lunch	Dinner	Bedtime		
			before / 1 hr. after	before / 1 hr. after	before / 1 hr. after			

Food

Breakfast	CHO	Portion	Lunch	CHO	Portion	Dinner	CHO	Portion
Snack	CHO	Portion	Snack	CHO	Portion	Snack	CHO	Portion

Exercise

Type		Duration

Comments

Day	Time	Insulin Dose/Type	Blood Glucose Test				Urine Ketone Tests	Notes
			Breakfast	Lunch	Dinner	Bedtime		
			before / 1 hr. after	before / 1 hr. after	before / 1hr. after			

Food

Breakfast		Lunch		Dinner		
CHO	Portion	CHO	Portion	CHO	Portion	
Snack		Snack		Snack		
CHO	Portion	CHO	Portion	CHO	Portion	

Exercise

Type	Duration

Comments

124

Day	Time	Insulin Dose/Type	Blood Glucose Test					Urine Ketone Tests	Notes
			Breakfast	Lunch	Dinner	Bedtime			
			before / 1 hr. after	before / 1 hr. after	before / 1 hr. after				

Food

Breakfast	CHO	Portion	Lunch	CHO	Portion	Dinner	CHO	Portion
Snack	CHO	Portion	Snack	CHO	Portion	Snack	CHO	Portion

Exercise

Type		Duration

Comments

Comparison of American and Canadian Food Group Systems

American Diabetes Association Exchange System		Canadian Diabetes Association Choice System
1 Starch	=	1 Starchy Foods
1 Lean Meat	=	1 Protein Foods
1 Medium-Fat Meat	=	1 Protein + 1/2 Fats & Oils
1 High-Fat Meat	=	1 Protein + 1 Fats & Oils
1 Vegetable	=	1/2 Fruits & Vegetables
(no equivalent)	=	Extra Vegetables
1 Fruit	=	1 1/2 Fruits & Vegetables
1 Milk	=	2 Milk (Skim)
1 Fat	=	1 Fats & Oils

Canadian Diabetes Association
Comparison of American and Canadian food group systems.
Diabetes Dialogue, 1988; 35 (4):57.

Index